FUE IN 7 DAYS

A FUE HAIR TRANSPLANT EXPERIENCE

Brian Martin

This non fiction book is a detailed account of the author's experience during the day of his FUE Hair Transplant and the 6 days that followed.

DEDICATION

**Dedicated to those who suffer from
inferiority issues due to hair loss.**

CONTENTS

DISCLAIMER

The author is not a doctor, nurse or any type of medical personal and does not have knowledge of medicine or any sort of knowledge of professional medical terms or procedures. This book is not to be treated as a professional medical reference or manual and should be treated exclusively as a personal account of the procedure, called a FUE Hair Transplant, that was performed on the author, as a patient, in Turkey, from the author's point of view and experience.

Should the reader go forward with any type of similar procedures as described in this book, the reader understands that in no way can the reader assume that the procedure described in this book will be the same, or will not change due to the course of time, that medications provided at the time of writing will not change or the results will be the same should the reader take on a similar procedure and the reader assumes all risks involved in taking such a procedure.

The author and events depicted in this book are entirely the author's personal experience. Any similarity to other events or persons, living or dead, is purely coincidental.

FOREWORD

First of all I want to thank you for purchasing this book. I am very sure that this information will be very valuable to anyone who is currently looking for information regarding FUE Hair transplants. It may help those looking for further information regarding this procedure. This book is composed from a journal of what I had written in during the first 7 days of having a FUE Hair Transplant procedure in Turkey.

It took me over a year to complete simply because I have included a series of week by week photos that clearly show the result up to a year after the operation in Istanbul, Turkey. The information gathered in this book is a very personal experience and whilst all of it is true, one needs to bear in mind that each case may be individual.

Readers should be aware that procedures may change over time due to modernisation of equipment, further scientific research and other things. I cannot take any responsibility for things that change over time, such as medications provided, new procedures implemented due to modernisation of any of the steps of the process or for any results or change in hotels and hospitals. In no way am I suggesting that anyone should have such a procedure and you understand that this is a personal choice and a personal risk.

What is written in here is just a personal account of what happened during the first 7 days during my personal experience of going through with a FUE hair transplant together with a series of photos of the results I achieved during the 51 weeks that followed. Furthermore, I added a little note about my progress after 365 days in the final chapter.

Knowing it is impossible to try and stop the illegal copying and sharing of such content over the internet, I do ask you to please respect the work I have put into this simple yet informative book. I decided to write and publish such a book because when I was looking for such information, it was not fully available in such a concise yet informative manner. Most of the information I required was either unavailable or hard to find through hundreds and hundreds of posts over a vast amount of online forums. However whilst some of the information was correct, most of it was speculative and instead of helping, complicated things further. A lot of detailed information has been included in this in the least possible manner.

The photos took much time to prepare and adapt to include in this book. That alone was a weekly process that a lot of time not only to take the photos every week, but also prepare them for publication. Use of photos on any other media is not permitted without my permission.

Therefore it is kindly appreciated that you share, not the book, but the link where one can purchase the book should they need to.

Thank You.

INTRODUCTION

At the time of writing this book I was 45 years old, I am now 46. This is not the first time I have written a short book, but I never imagined that I would be writing a book about a hair transplant experience, let alone writing a book about my own experience. I have been suffering from hair loss since I was in my early twenties and each year that would go by I would see less and less hair covering my head. In 2006, when I turned 33 I decided to shave my hair completely. I could not bear to see myself in the mirror the first time I shaved my hair and decided to grow it back on. Sadly after a few months I had to give in to the fact and reality of the situation that my residing hair was now in an advanced stage and shaved it again.

In all honesty it took me quite a while to get used to the image I kept seeing in front of the mirror. Image was very important to me because I work in an industry where you are in a spotlight most of the time when at work, the business of show business. Being a focal point most of the time, in front of hundreds of people makes a person very conscious of their appearance. Needless to say, this affected me physiologically.

In my mind, it didn't matter if people preferred me with hair or not, if I looked good with no hair and it made no difference when people told me I looked good as I was. Knowing I was balding did not make me feel good and subconsciously it was affecting my life, both work-wise and at home. It created a sense of insecurity , inferiority, and unfortunately an unreal perception. This is not an uncommon feeling among men, who for most of their early life would have had hair to be proud of and then start seeing their hairline recede.

As a man, the worst thing was knowing that not everyone is the same, some men go bald fast once the initial process kicks in, others loose hair at a slower pace and others don't have to worry about it. According to a recent scientific study I read somewhere, it was proven that hair does make a man look more attractive to the majority of people, however bald man are perceived as more mature, wiser and in some cases sexier. But tell that to someone who has not accepted and embraced the fact that they are balding and most will tell you that they don't feel that way and feel that something has been stolen.

I too felt that something was stolen from me and whether this was just my hair, it did reflect my youth and my image. Whatever it was, made no no difference. I just felt naked and thought people would perceive me as such. If all bald or balding men are like me, they would all think that everyone is looking at, or thinking about, their residing hair. In reality this is not so and the only person that actually cares is the person balding!

In all honesty, I only realised this after having my transplant because it was then that I realised that it really does not make a difference to have or not have hair. After having had the transplant, I started telling people and almost everyone told me that I seemed good the way I way I was, except one person and that was my mother. She was the only person who told me that I look better with hair than without and surprisingly she was very happy about it. Now if there is one person who is, and should be, honest with me is my mother. So I am quite happy that I did actually have the transplant, especially since the process is proving to be a success as you will see in the photos.

The journey is now an ongoing process now over 12 months old and I am quite happy that I got most of my hair back and I do admit that for me, it really does make a difference to my life. However the initial stages are very slow, but eventually those buds start sprouting and eventually they get longer and with it comes a sense of security and and sense of feeling better.

Ironically, the idea of writing a book about my experience came to me while on the operating chair. You will understand why I call it a chair later on in this book. I had 8 hours to think of things and the thoughts that came to me during the operation were quite odd, but surprisingly good. You would think that during such a surgery one's mind would be stressed or obsessed about the procedure, but this only occurred to me during the first 50-70mins of the operation and once those passed, then I was left with plenty of time to think of many other things, one of them was writing this book about my experience. However I did not just want it to be a book about hair transplants, but a book describing my experience with informative details about the surgery and post surgery I personally experienced, which I believe is a unique experience to each and every individual.

The idea began as a 7 day journal of my experience but later on I decided to also include photos of the results achieved during the 51 weeks that followed, making developing it into a 12 month story, part in photographic detail. Of course I wanted to release my book sooner than the year ahead, mainly to help those who are intending to take a leap, but time is time and things had to take their course. Now I feel the wait was worth it and the book offers a more detailed account with the set of photos of the results.

My experience actually commenced a few months before the operation, when I saw an advert that caught my attention on Facebook. It was about having an FUE transplant in Turkey. For some strange reason it caught my attention and even though I had given in to the idea of reaming bald and shaving for the rest of my life, I clicked on the ad and was served with a website that promoted FUE hair transplants in Istanbul, Turkey at a very affordable cost.

I researched a little online found out more about FUE transplants, but not enough information about having it done in Turkey. Actually some of the forums I visited had several posts that put off other people from having hair transplants done in Turkey, but never were these posts based on their own personal experience. I now presume that most people would imagine Turkey as some sort of undeveloped country, but I had visited Istanbul over 10 times before and I knew that there are quite technologically advanced in some areas more than others. However I was still a little weary about it after reading some of the posts in the forum, so I thought no more of it at that point.

Then as if by destiny's calling, a few days after my visit to the hair restoration site, I met a friend whom I had not seen for quite some time and noticed his pinkish hairs and tell tail signs of a very recent FUE transplant. I took the courage to ask him if he had done anything to his hair and he told me that he had done a FUE hair transplant, guess where? He gave me a very brief and vague idea of his experience, the hotel, the clinic but not too much information about what I was really expecting to hear. I did ask him if it was painful and he told me no it wasn't at all, except the local anaesthetic injections they inject in your head to numb the area they perform surgery on, but compared it the type of pain you receive from a dentist's injection!

My brief encounter geared me up to search a little more that evening and eventually I got in contact through the website that popped up as an advert on Facebook a few days earlier and received a reply from a guy called Kaan. The responses and correspondence was very courteous and professional throughout and after sending photos of the current situation of my hair I received a free online consultation, directly from the surgeon, informing me of what can and what could not be done for me. Here is the consultation I received:

"Mr. Martin is an ideal candidate for an FUE technique hair transplant operation. With his donor region, we can offer him a full coverage around all the thinning and bald patches at the front and top areas in one session completely and obtain a good hairline level with a very dense look permanently, which matches the rest of his current hair. For the crown, I am explaining what we can offer below as well.

As the first thing to do, we will bring Patient' s temples and frontal hairline back by forming to its original shape and follow the current receded frontal hairline, considering the patient's age and visage as well. We will show this in front of a mirror and decide together for the level. The density we will be reaching would be between 36 to 40 Grafts per cm2 at the front, offering him a good dense looking hair at the front for styling.

Following this, we will continue implanting the healthy hair follicles backwards and cover all the top area with a good density of 30-32 grafts per cm2. Again, when implanting, we will use the grafts wisely and place them with different angles to get the best natural look for the future.

Crown area: As Mr. Martin's donor region is not enough to cover the crown completely, I can only use the rest of the hairs harvested to increase the density a bit. But, it won't be like the front or top unfortunately. Therefore, if he definitely wants a full coverage, he might use fibre involving products such as Toppik or equivalents. On the day of the operation, I will try my best to harvest more than I suggest him without leaving any patchy look at the back. So he is looking for a 65 - 70% coverage in total.

We will implant the hair follicles with a variety of angles, achieving a 100% natural look with 3000+ Grafts (~7000 hairs) and the patient' s donor area is good enough to harvest this amount.

I forecast a successful operation and a fast recovery for the patient."

I was intrigued by the idea and decided to proceed with the whole thing and my journey began there and then. I was scheduled to fly to Istanbul within a month and a half after my initial contact with Kaan and the hair surgeon but time flew past fast.

As the day was approaching, insecurities started to set in again. I was getting more nervous on each passing day, worrying about if I had made the right decision, thinking to myself that it is still not too late and I can turn back and all I would have lost was the deposit I had paid. I had many restless and sleepiness night prior to the day I had to depart, thinking of the worst that could happen. I also was wondering if I was making the right decision because I had to block work for at least two weeks, that meant no money coming in and no guarantee that I would be fit to face any audience once the two suggested recovery weeks were up.

However the idea of regaining my hair seemed to have won over the negative thoughts and eventually the day came when I had to travel to Istanbul. This is was the day where my experience really begun and it is from here that I will leave you to experience my procedure the way I remember it during those first 7 days of having my FUE Hair Transplant done in Turkey.

DAY 1
9TH APRIL

This was the day I have been waiting for now for almost two months from my initial contact with Mr Kaan. I Started off in the morning with a herbal tea, remembering that coffee was not recommended for a few days prior to the operation. Kaan had provided me with a set of instructions and things I needed for my short visit to Turkey. Although I had been preparing everything for two weeks, I still was packing three hours before leaving for the airport for my three day life changing experience in Istanbul. I must admit that I received a little help from my girlfriend who made sure to prepare the clothes I needed the night before.

Finally it was time to drive to the airport, again my girlfriend took on that shore and we arrived right on time, safely of course. Checking in and boarding the plane, Turkish Airlines, was no hassle at all. After experiencing Turkish Airlines for the first time I would defiantly recommend them to anyone. The journey was just a three hour flight and a comfortable one. The meals were the most enjoyable I had on a plane that I can remember in a long time. The plane landed safely in Istanbul and as soon as I was out of the plane and into the arrivals hall, to my surprise I was greeted by my personal assistant that guided me through the airport saving lots of time in the queues, a real relief. This is real VIP service. After passing immigration controls, which again was a very pleasant process, and making it out of the airport I was greeted by Mr Kaan. I had only communicated with Kaan via emails and over the phone and he always sounded professional, polite and courteous through these channels. The same could be said when meeting him face to face. He is truly a very nice professional person. We had a brief chat and Mr. Kann introduced me to my personal patient coordinator, Mr Adnan who guided me to the luxury vehicle awaiting me.

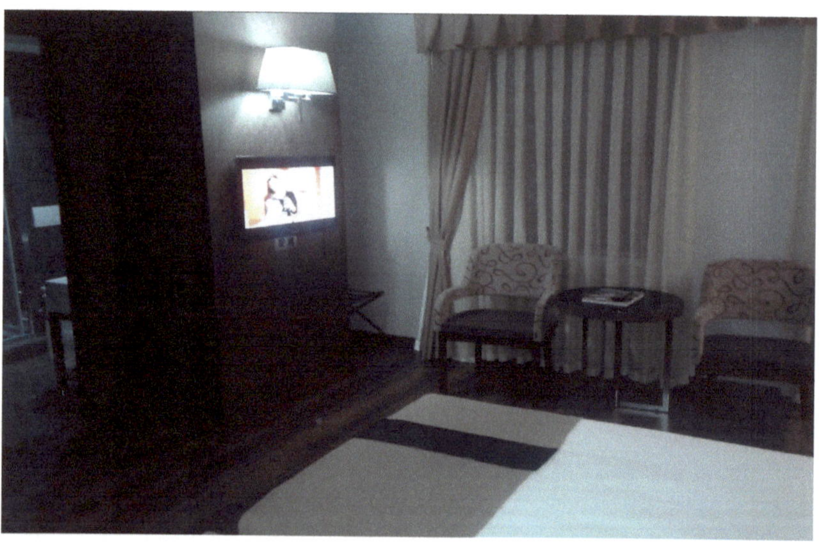

The hotel, actually a very nice 4 star hotel, was not far from the airport, about 30-40mins during rush hour, so if you arrive in Istanbul at another time I guess you would reach the hotel in less time. During the ride Mr Kaan explained and answered the little questions I had not asked before, reassuring me that I was about to get the best service possible and my choice was spot on. We arrived at the hotel and immediately checked in which was a simple 5min process. After checking in I was taken to my room which was better than what I expected, spotless clean and extremely modern and comfortable, exactly what one would expect during this kind of situation.

Again Mr Kaan detailed all the things I needed to do and prepare for the following morning and gave me a briefing of the next day leaving me to my own devices for the rest of evening and night to follow.

I decided to go down to the restaurant to have dinner and on the way down, in the elevator, I came face to face with two young men who that had just done the operation the day before. They were wearing headbands and I noticed some slightly blood stained bandages underneath at the back of their head, but my eyes could not stop starring at the implanted part on their head. It looked very painful and I was having second thoughts. However these guys were joking, laughing and didn't seem at all in pain as a matter of fact they looked extremely happy and content. Their faces said it all. I introduced myself to them and asked them if they had the FUE done, to which they had both confirmed. Then I told them that I was going to do it the following day and although bandaged they ensured me that they were not in any sort of pain.

The fact that people in the hotel are used to seeing bandaged guys with redness on top of their heads, running around the hotel, eased my worries about the impact this fact bared on me and provided me with the confidence I was lacking thinking of how I would approach the world after the op. For dinner I selected a lovely chicken dish, which apart from being very tasty was really good. I must say I love Turkish food and the way it is cooked. After dinner I decided to go out and have a quick stroll around the area the hotel was located in.

It was kind of late so the only shops open at the time were coffee shops, restaurants and of course the famous Turkish kebab shops. This was the real thing. I must say that the hotel is situated in quite a nice area, and although it is not a tourist area, I felt quite at home and very safe.

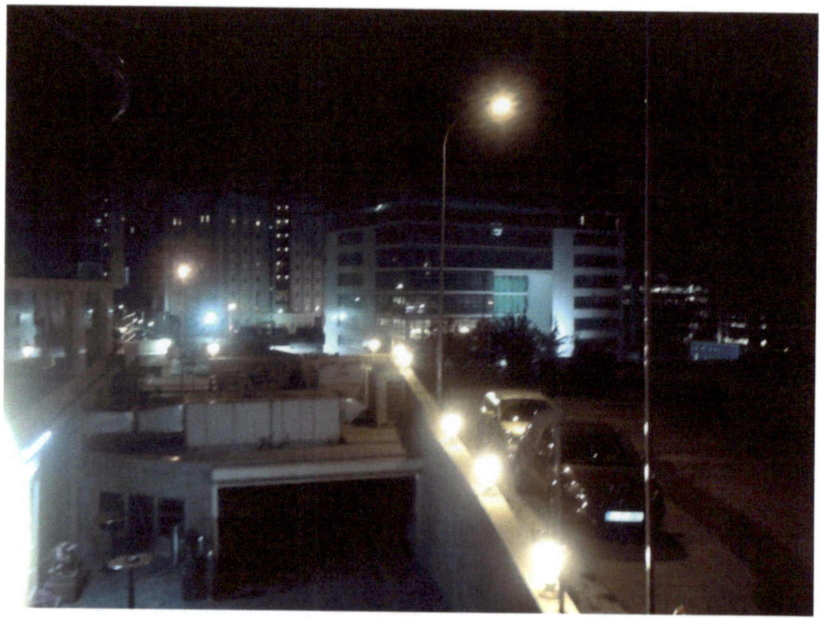

After around an hour strolling and discovering the surroundings, I felt it was time to return to the hotel to have a shower and to relax in order to prepare myself, mentally and physically, for the next day, the day of my op.

The nerves and the stress I had experienced for the past few weeks were now down to a level of almost zero. I was feeling very excited by the fact that after many years thinking about it, I had finally taken the plunge and thoughts and wishes of having the hair transplant done were now becoming a reality. After a nice shower I lay my head upon the soft pillow and must have fell asleep instantly.

DAY 2
10TH APRIL

After a really good sleep and a very comfortable night, I woke up a little earlier than usual, showered and went down for breakfast. Usually, when at home, my breakfast consists of coffee with either some toast and cheese, or crackers and cheese or cereal, depending on the mood I have woken up to. Don't ask me why, but when on holiday I like having a traditional English breakfast. The fact that it is prepared for you is perhaps the reason why I opt for this sort of thing and although not at all healthy it's delicious! Today I did completely the opposite and must admit that breakfast has been the healthiest I've ever had when located in a hotel abroad. Fruit, Turkish tea, orange juice and for the naughty bit a croissant.

During breakfast I noted another two young men on an adjacent table who appeared to have had the op performed the day before. These were not the same two men I met in the elevator the night before. I didn't get to speak with them though but they too seemed to be quite happy and relaxed. Considering that my op was now just a matter of hours away, I felt to have eased my nerves and felt no signs of tension and thoughts of what I was about to proceed with, later on that day, did not cross my mind.

The operation was scheduled at 3pm which meant that I had a whole morning to roam around the area and perhaps buy a little present for my girlfriend while exploring the place that will eventually give me back a little more confidence. I am now really looking forward to the process. So right after breakfast, I ventured off to explore the surrounding areas around the hotel, and perhaps window shop. Unfortunately, this area isn't much of a tourist area but mainly a business area, with the clinic being perhaps the main attraction, attracting medical tourism to the area. Although there were many shops, I did not purchase anything as nothing appealed to me which is quite unusual but I did stop at a cute little tea place or bread shop, they offered both, and had a lovely Turkish tea.

The kids serving me, in their early twenties, were ever so sweet. I relaxed a bit and savored the ambient of Istanbul, people going around their daily business and doing their thing. Kaan was to collect me at 2pm, but it was only just 11am and I still had plenty of time on my hands with nothing else to do so I decided to go back to the hotel to have a rest before the op. The hotel was only about a 10 minute walk away from where I was, 3 of which were spent trying to cross the busy Turkish roads.

Back at the hotel I contacted my girlfriend over Skype. I was wishing that she was here but at the same time after seeing all the men who were coming here alone for their ops, I was quite content we decided that it would perhaps be better for her not to come. It could have been quite a traumatic event for her, especially the first night after the op. Therefore based on my experience, it would be much better to go alone or to go with a friend, perhaps someone who is interested in doing the same process themselves than going with a spouse or partner unless you plan to spend a few more days prior to or after the op.

The hotel is equipped with good WIFI and after feeling rather bored going through FB, having checked my emails and chatting to my girlfriend, I decided to wait for Kaan downstairs in the lobby, an hour ahead of the planned time. While downstairs in the lobby, I met up with the two guys I had spoken to in the elevator and yet another young man, from Lebanon, who had the op performed just as I was arriving at the hotel the previous evening together with the other two men I saw during breakfast.

"Right!", I thought to myself, "Seems like I'm not the only one who wanted to get back what I had lost!" They further encouraged me that they were fine and were not in any sort of pain, the only drawback, they explained, was the uncomfortable feeling when trying to get some sleep. I then received a very good tip from the guy from Lebanon. He told me that the only thing he wished he had done after the op was go to sleep before the local anesthetic had worn off. It was there and then that I decided to take his advice and I am happy to relay this advice to anyone who decides to go ahead with this procedure.

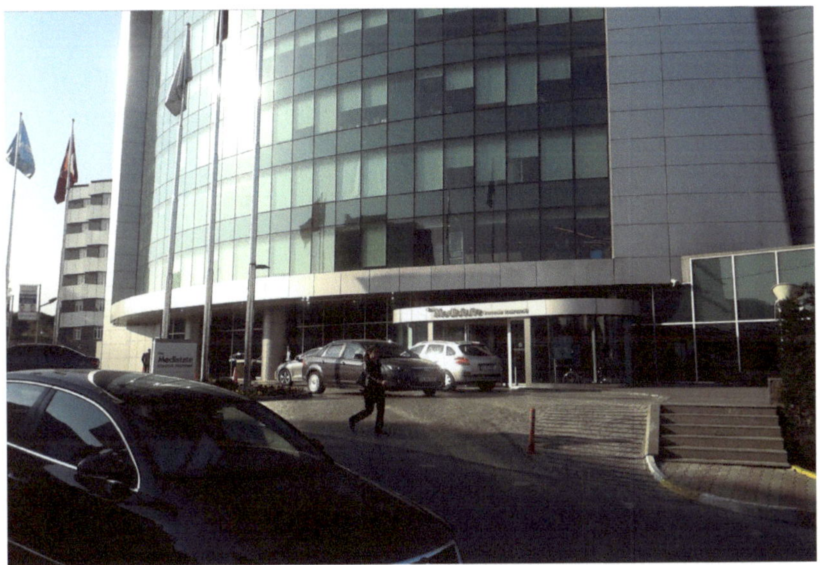

At 2pm Kaan came to pick me up from the hotel , as promised, to take me to the clinic, Medistate Clinic. The hotel is only a few minutes away from the hotel by foot and a little more than that time by car. I did mention the traffic didn't I?

The service given was a 5 star service, as I was guided into the clinic and taken up to the 8th floor, where the op was going to be performed.

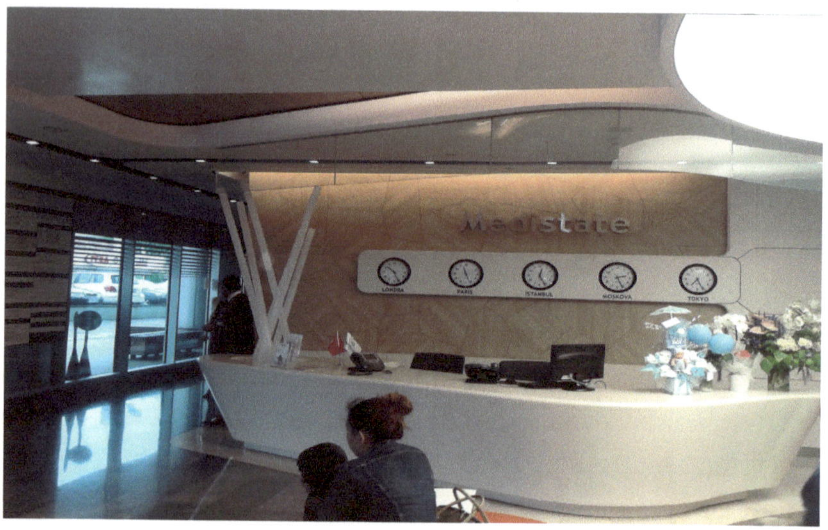

Being greeted by all the staff calmed me and eased my nerves that were now beginning to mount up at a steady speed. I was introduced to the medical team and then the surgeon, Dr Tofun Oguzoglu and a lady who not only spoke my language but also very good English acted as a translator. The surgeon spoke very good English as well, but some of the other nurses were not so conversant in English.

After examining my donor hair he discovered that I had a better donor area than what he thought I did when he saw the photos I had supplied during my online consultation with Kaan. So he decided that for a good result he was able to provide me, about 3500 in one session, enough to cover my hairline and top surface area. The only thing missing would then be hair on my small crown, but this is something that I could either cover or have transplanted in a separate op 12 months from my initial transplant, should I wish to.

The surgeon was also content to note that apart from having a good donor area, the donor hair was thick, a good sign he said because it would give me density which would provide for me an 80% total coverage. The other 20% would be spread around the transplant, the donor area and the small crow, the small crown being the most part uncovered. I was hoping he would be able to cover the small crown as well in the same op, since this was the first place to go when I started loosing hair, but I still was not disappointed with the final outcome of the pre op examination. After all I had been without a small crown for many years before the rest f it started straying away from my head.

I was then led to the op theater, where I changed into the usual medical jacket, however unlike other ops, I was allowed to keep my jeans and also use a mobile phone for entertainment purposes, though I opted not to in the beginning. My blood pressure and blood samples were taken, they need it to check for sugar levels and other things and my head was shaved and cleaned ready for the op. A short while after my head was cleaned, the surgeon entered to mark the places from where the donor hair was to be taken with his pen. Once this procedure was over, I was asked to sit on the operating chair. I call it an operating chair because that is what it appeared to be to me, a chair that could be compared to a dentist chair/massage parlor table. This was the part I was dreading because this was the part that most people online complained about, the local anesthetic injected into the scalp.

After several injections around the donor area, which I would not call painless, but neither would I call painful, the surgeon checked if the area to be worked on was in fact numb. It was. The chair was then receded making it a bed and I was then asked to turn face down. As soon as I was in a comfortable position, the surgeon began the process of extracting the initial follicles to examine them under the lens. When extracting them a small drill is used with a specialised bit that is just short of being 1mm in diameter. Each follicle is drilled and then is extracted by being pulled with a tweezers, I think. I say I think because that is exactly what it felt like, but I could not see since I was face down and they were tacking the lower back of my head.

After the surgeon examined the initial 10s of follicles extracted, the nurses took over to extract all that could be safely extracted from the donor area, leaving it looking as natural as possible. The surgeon was happy to announce that I still had a good amount of hair in the donor area with each follicle containing an average of about 2.5 hairs, meaning most follicles contained 3 grafts, whilst the second was 2 grafts and quite a few containing 4 grafts. This means that less donor extractions was required in order to provide me with about 3500 grafts that were needed. The nurses took over 2 hours to extract the donor hair and the process was indeed painless.

During the extraction process one will experience the slightest of all tugs during the harvesting of the donor hairs, but this would be impossible to eliminate completely. Nevertheless it is painless. As soon as the harvesting is completed, the donor area is then washed and cleaned and I was then asked to turn around and sit up slowly. More cleaning of the area was done and the area was bandaged up immediately. The nurses asked me if I was feeling OK and gave me a small fruit juice in order to replenish any sugar level lost during the extraction process. My blood pressure was once again taken and a green light was given for the incision, or graft, process which is conducted personally by the surgeon. To be noted is that the time between harvesting and implanting is crucial during all moments of the process. The least time between these two process means a successful process. Therefore the surgeon must be capable of grafting precisely, swiftly and artfully.

This is after all a cosmetic surgery, therefore the cosmetics must look realistic. This is why a surgeon with both artistic, swift and with a good medical background is required for any successful Hair Transplant. Thee surgeon came in and proceeded with constructing my hairline using a laser assisted piece of equipment. He then went on to draw the hairline he could acquire and showed me the resulting output for approval before commencing the grafting process. For the incisions, I was seated upright at an angle of about 75 degrees, comfortable enough for the surgeon to be able to work on me. Then the nurses commenced numbing the areas the surgeon would be working upon using local anesthetic once again.

If you are wondering if this numbing process is painful, then I will be honest and tell you that this is definitely the most painful part of the whole process and if you want something to compare the pain with, then you can compare the feeling to that of being injected by a dentist. It is still quite difficult to compare, since I had been to different dentists some of which involved a rather painful injection and others where had if I been blindfolded I would not have realised that I had been injected. For comparison on a scale of 1 -10, 10 being the most painful dentist and 1 being the most delicate dentist I would scale these injection to the scalp at about 5-6. As soon at the local anesthetic was applied the grafting process begun, 3300 grafts, each swiftly but precisely applied in order to create a natural flow of hair. In some other countries law does not oblige surgeons to perform the grafts but obliges them to supervise the process. However in Turkey, this part of the process has to performed exclusively by the surgeon as required by the laws of the country. This may perhaps be one of the best advantages of having any kind of cosmetic surgery there.

The whole process must have taken between 1hr to 1.15hrs and although I still have no idea how the counting was conducted, I had other things on my mind at that moment, I assume that the surgeon would be counting 100 grafts at a time and then he would briefly stop for a few seconds to dab the areas away from any blood. I did however note that during each of these stops, one of the nurses said something in Turkish, this I think were total amount of grafts performed for each small pause. So she could have been counting too.

Once the grafting process was completed, my scalp was cleaned and I was once again asked to slowly sit upright. Every one asked me if was feeling OK and if I should feel any dizziness to inform them. But I was feeling fine, a little jammed due to the long period seated. I would compare the process as being seated on a long flight without being able to move unless instructed to while someone is playing with your head. Now the nurses came to give me some good news, that I was allowed a very short break, enough time to use the bathroom and have a small snack consisting of a burger and juice.

Surprisingly I felt quite hungry and the snack did actually prepare me for the next and final process, that of implanting the hairs into the grafts. I would recommend using the bathroom because the next process is long, without any breaks. After my short 15min break I was back on the surgical chair (I think this is a more justifying name for the chair) in the same position as I was a short while back while grafts were being made by the surgeon. The process commenced almost immediately, with two nurses, one on either side, performing the painstaking job of inserting a single hair in each graft.

During the time I decided to Skype text my girlfriend, to notify her that I was doing well and undergoing the last process, which was scheduled to last for about 2.5hrs. This was a good idea as after testing I then decided to read an e book I had downloaded on my phone and been meaning to read for quite a while. I also was brave enough to take a selfie!

The nurses consistently performed their painstaking job and every now and again the surgeon would enter to take a look at the work performed by them and evaluate it. I decided to try and count the number of times each nurse implanted a hair per minute.

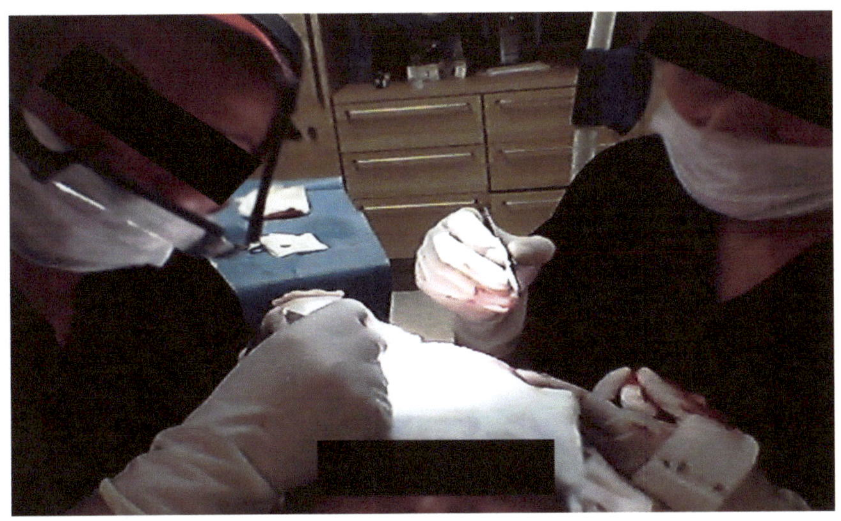

The nurse on my left hand side was doing about 9 per minute, the nurse on my right hand side was doing about 7 per minute. After about 2.15hrs the nurse on the left had finished her job, the nurse on the right had still few more to implant but was ready 15mins after. Finally the words I wanted to hear came our of the nurse's mouth. Sir you are ready. A sense of freedom overcome with joy and relief spread through my body, Finally I was done. I took a quick look at my watch and it was about 9:40pm. My eight hour ordeal was finally over, sort of. I still had another 20 minutes to go.

First I was helped up, asked if I felt OK and as soon as I asserted that I was good I was gently cleaned from the blood that covered some parts of my scalp. Until that point I was completely calm throughout the operation, however there was one part that I was dreading, that of the extraction of the intravenous needle from my right arm. You should know that I hate needles and I can´t stand the sight or thought of blood. I hate having blood extracted from me and I feel faint with even the thought of it. So I made sure that the nurses and patient coordinators knew about this before so that when this moment arrives they would know what to expect from me. I was not looking at the process making sure to turn my sight in the other direction. The nurse obviously noticing that I was petrified, instead of pulling off the plaster that was fixing the apparatus to my veins, decided to use alcohol to dampen the plaster to reduce the stickiness so that I will not feel it as much. I felt the tugging on the plaster and at the same time the spray of the alcohol on my arm and screamed out thinking that the nurse had extracted the needle and blood was spraying all over the place. Everyone was suddenly in shock as I was was shouting out "Blood, blood, blood everywhere!!". The nurse was in turn replying, "No blood Sir, no blood, only alcohol, no blood". My reply, "Yes blood, blood!".

After about 30 seconds of this charade, I turned my head expecting to see blood streaming out of my veins and everywhere covered in it but to my surprise I saw a clean hand and the nurse with a spray gun in her hand containing the cleaning alcohol liquid. This was a scene from one of those black comedy films and it was there that I burst out laughing at the situation. Taking advantage of the appropriate time, the nurse took the opportunity to take out the needle swiftly and plaster the small wound without me even noticing.

I guess this was the funniest moment of the whole process and the one everyone in that room would remember me for.

The nurses then went on to take off the surgical jacket they had supplied me with and help me put on my top and shoes. I was once again given a drink and was led out to the reception area. That could very well be the last time I saw or set foot in that operating theatre, at least for 12 months or more so I took one good last look at it and secretly said goodbye to it.

At the reception area the Melanie, the English speaking lady from Tunis, explained in detail what I had to do next. I was supplied with a sweatband that was placed over my forehead and which I was to keep on for the following three days.

A number of medications and treatments, including antibiotics and painkillers and a special lotion and shampoo, were also given to me. I have listed these all below together with the doses prescribed and photos.

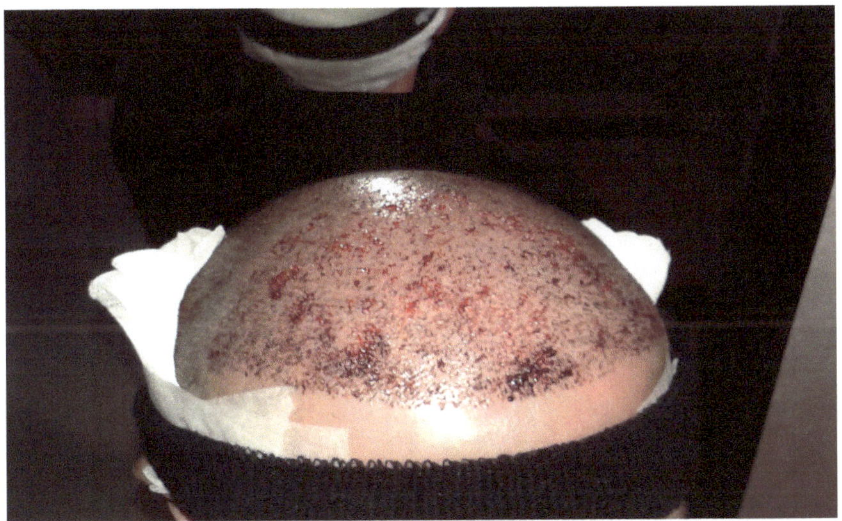

The painkillers were only given in the case if I felt pain, once the effects of the anesthetic wore off. I was also instructed on how to sleep for the first couple of nights, face upwards without tuning to the sides. The sweatband was there for two reasons, one was to keep the bandage adhered to the back of my head and the other was to keep the swelling from not spreading to other parts of my face. Also a special cover, a protective baby changing sheet, for the pillow was given to me and so was a surgical hat that was placed on me and which had to be taken off as soon as I reached my room. Once all the briefing was done, I was then accompanied to the private vehicle waiting outside the clinic ready to take me back to the hotel.

The weather had changed outside and it was raining when I exited the clinic. Luckily the vehicle was just at the clinic's door so this did not effect me and Adnan was by my side with the umbrella. Within a few minutes I was at the hotel, from where I left earlier that afternoon. By now it was about 10:30pm. The receptionists at the hotel are obviously used to seeing patients entering after just getting a hair transplant and other cosmetic operations, so it was no shock or surprise to them seeing me enter wearing the surgical cap.

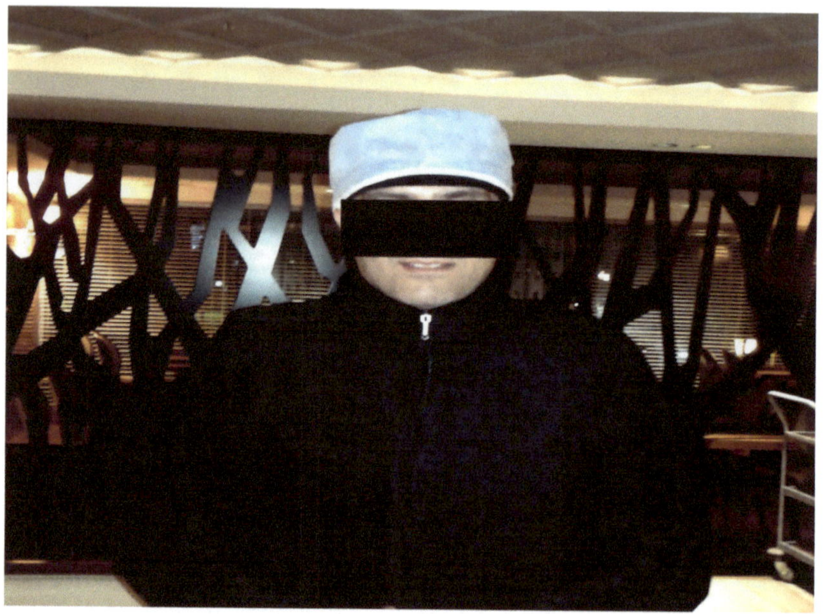

I was accompanied by the clinic's patient coordinator, Adnan and Kaan through out the whole time. I needed to eat something in order to commence taking the medicine that was supplied so I ordered a burger from the restaurant below and asked for it to be delivered to my room. We then went up to my room and once there Kaan and Adnan ensured that I was OK and that everything was good. Kaan briefed me about what to expect next, slight pain once the anesthetic wears off, most probably a slight discomfort when trying to lie down and some numbness in some areas and before leaving me for the night scheduled to collect me the following day at 12.30pm. When they left I was tempted to remove the cap to see the workings but decided not to do so until my food was delivered as I did not wish to scare the poor man delivering my food. Food came within 10mins and I ate most of it because I wasn't really hungry just needed something before in order to take the antibiotics and anti-inflammatory tablets I was supplied with so that they start working by the time the numbing effect wears off. After eating, I took the medicine provided and got changed, keeping in mind the advice given to me earlier in the morning to try to get to sleep before the effect of the anesthetic wore off.

Taking off my t-shirt was easy as it was a little stretchy and I wore it intentionally to make the process easy. I covered the pillow with the protective cover given to me at the clinic and laid on my back instructed I used a very good method to sleep instantly and to not keep my mind working on the experience I had just been through. The method is something that puts me to sleep within 8mins flat. It is actually an audio course I had bought and uploaded to my phone. I have been trying to listen to this course for over 6 months though, but always manage to fall asleep after about 7mins, since the person's voice does a very good job a putting me to sleep whenever I hear it on my headphones. It may not have thought me anything about the course as I never get past the introduction but it does a pretty good job in putting me to sleep, so I use it quite often. During the night I woke up a couple of times, each time expecting some pain or discomfort, but experienced neither of the two and just replayed the mp3 to which I slept again until the following morning. Considering everything I do have a fairly good night's sleep.

The list of medicinals and the dosage prescribed are as will follow.

Please note, I am not describing what they are and what they do because I would like you to search for them yourselves online. Do not ask me either, because the information online can give you a better explanation of what they are for, what side effects they could have and who can and who cannot take them.

The items listed and the dosage given are exclusive information I could not find shared anywhere else. Also note that the medicines and/or the dosages prescribed to me may have been exclusive to my needs and requirements and may be very different to what is needed to be provided to anyone else.

Warning

Do not take any of the medicines described on the next pages unless advised and prescribed by a licensed medical doctor. I am only listing this to give you a one ahead advantage in case you suffer from any allergies or medical conditions that prevent you form using the medicinals below, before these are given to you on the day and I assume no liability should anyone decide to try these based on what is written below.

Before taking any medicine, patients should check with their doctors who should provide a proper prescription.

The following is what was prescribed to me, medicinals, kits and dosage:

Lansor: 30mg 1 daily x 6days

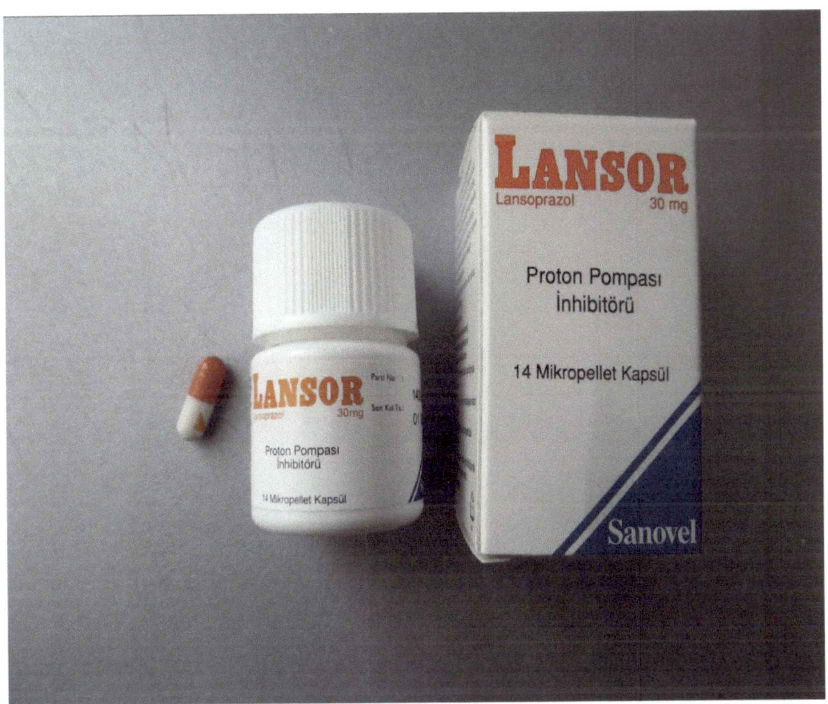

Prendol: 16mg x 6days.

 1st day x 3 tablets to be taken at the same time,

2nd day x 3 tablets at the same time,

3rd day x 2 tablets at the same time,

4th day x 2 tablets at the same time,

5th day x 1 tablet

6th day x 1 tablet

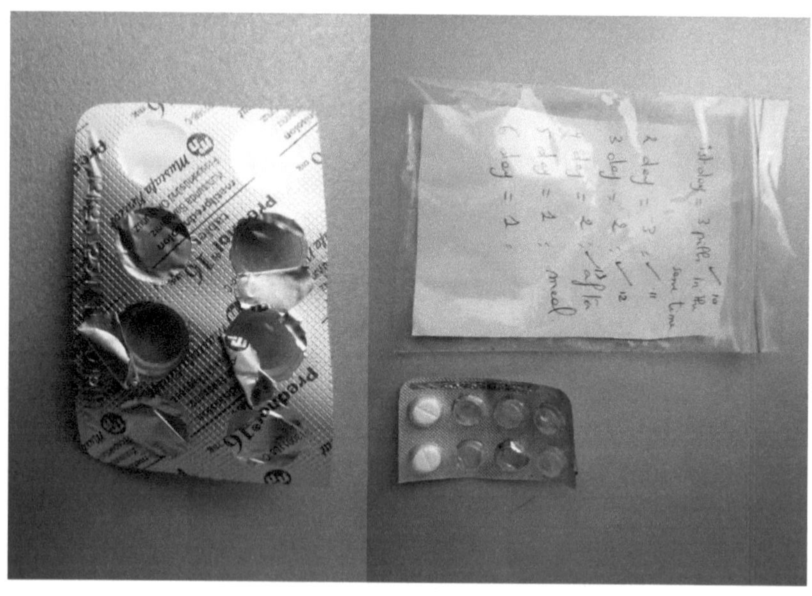

Tetradox: 2 x daily 1 morning, 1 night.

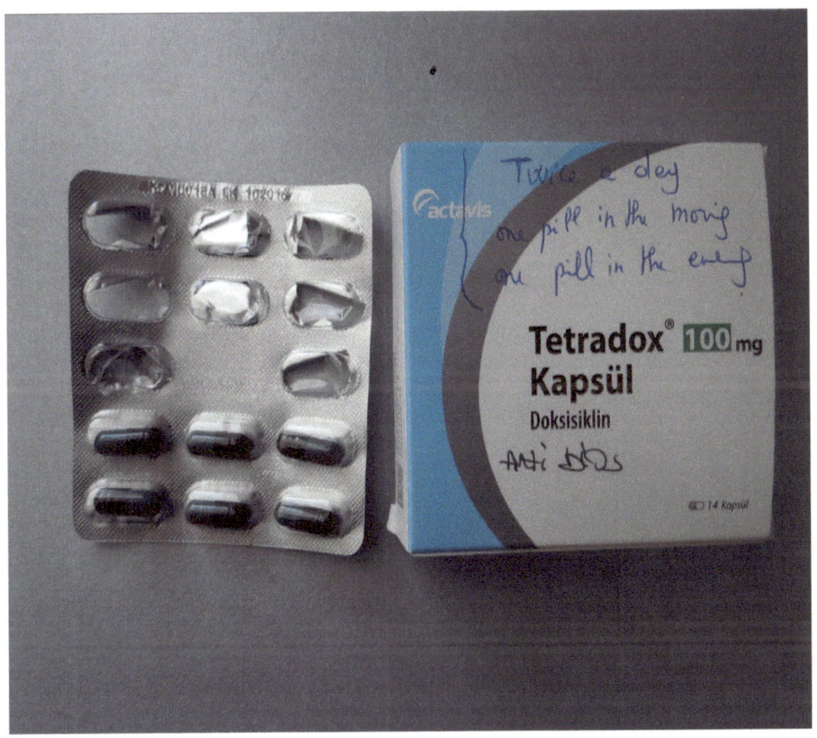

Hairixin Hair Transplant Kit:

Usage 1 time daily x 15days.

Use cream to cover implants, patting in cream gently, Leave it in for 30mins,

Rinse cream with lukewarm water.

Shampoo all head and rinse with lukewarm water.

Do not rub in, pat gently.

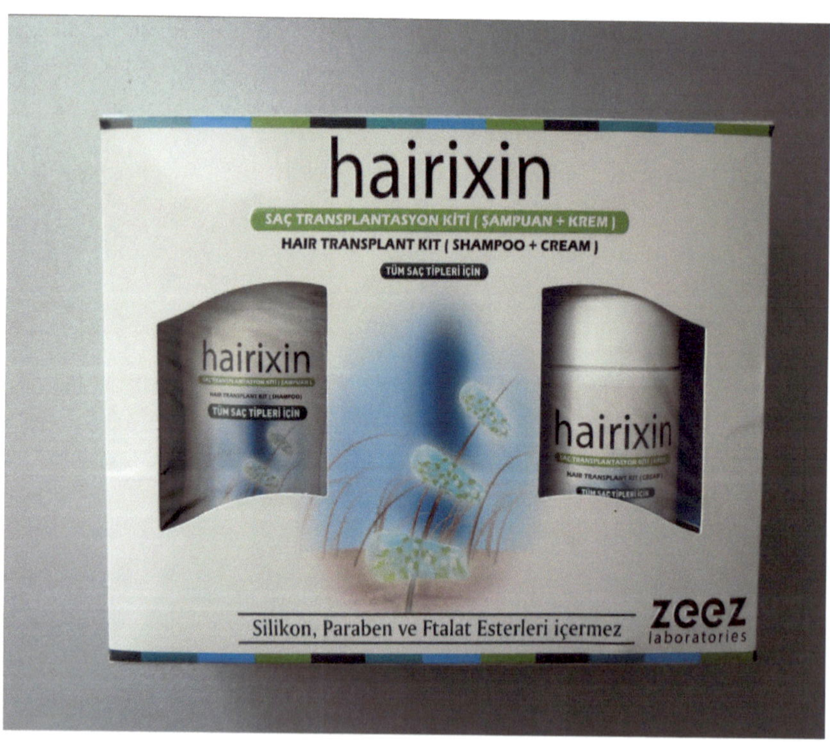

DAY 3
11TH APRIL

Amazingly despite the long ordeal of the day before, I woke up early but slept well enough considering the sequence of events yesterday. The first thing I did after getting up from bed was to check the pillow and sheets for signs of blood and was expecting to see much of it, but to my surprise there was only minimal signs on the cover that was placed on the pillow. Next I went straight to the the mirror and looked to see what my head looked like this fine morning.

I cannot say that I liked what I saw as I can only compare what I saw to a beetroot. My head looked a quite red and a bit swollen but overall I guess it is looked much better compared to some photos I had found and seen on the internet of other operations. I was expecting the swelling as I had read about this prior to the operation.

Apparently swelling occurs due to a liquid that is injected in the scalp to facilitate the process for the surgeon and nurses. I know about this liquid because I once read an news feature about Gordon Ramsay's hair transplant op since his face swelled due to the liquid spreading. I was told not to wash my head, so obviously avoided that when showering and soon after dressed to go down for breakfast.

I felt a bit odd during breakfast, odd in a way that I felt everyone was looking at me, but in reality no one seemed to care. I still tried to stay to the side as much as possible in order to not disgust anyone who may be having breakfast, I know that I could not bear the site myself had it been the other way around. I took my morning pill but I did not go out or do much after breakfast and just waited in my room until it was time to be collected to go and visit the clinic so that they can undress the bandaging, cleanse the scalp and the area where the extraction took place and show me how to take care of it once I am alone at home.

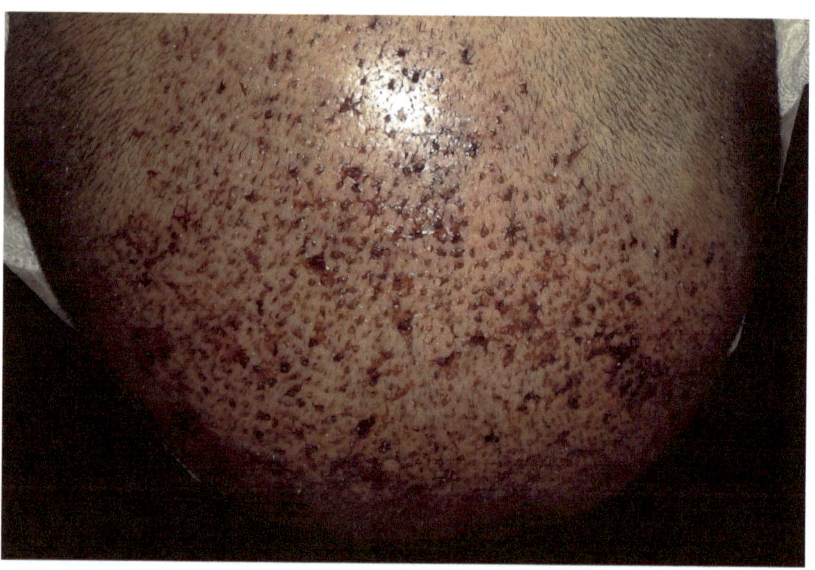

As usual Adnan, the patient coordinator, came right on time and took me to the clinic where, as expected, I was instructed on how to apply the lotion and use the shampoo, part of the hair transplant kit provided (as described above). The nurse showed me through the process for the first time. She applied the cream lotion and that stood on for 30mins.

Once 30mins had passed I was taken into another room with a

sink and there they took off my bandage from the back of my head. While the nurse was doing this I felt a burning sensation, as the bandage was slightly adhered to the skin due to the drying blood that came out from the previous night. While it was being gently pulled off I felt it since the skin was still extremely sensitive due to the process of extraction the previous night.

Apart from that,   no other pains were experienced, just a slight tingle wherever my head would be rinsed with water. The lotion was then rinsed with lukewarm water and my whole head was then shampooed with the special shampoo.

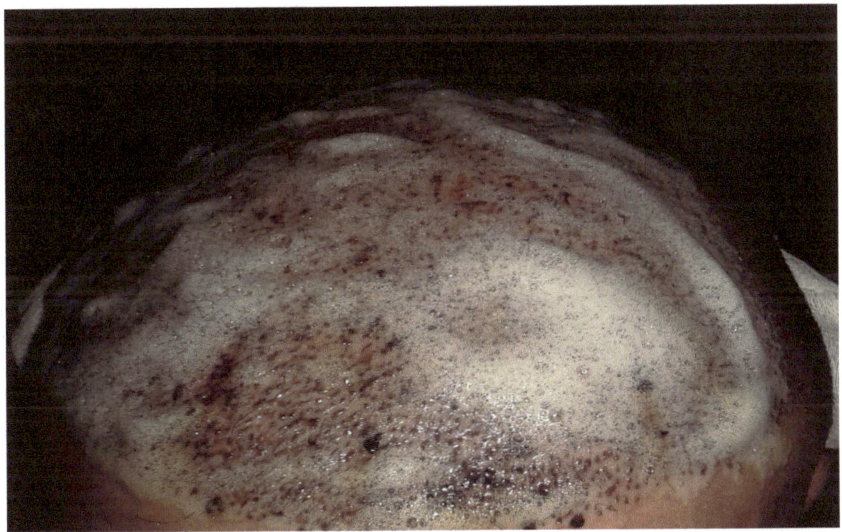

My head was then kitchen towel dried, the process is done by gently tapping several pieces of paper towel until the head was no longer wet. A quick inspection of the process by the nurses and consultant,(the surgeon had already flew to Dubai for another operation there) and every looked very good according to them. The back of my head was re-bandaged and I was given a funny cap to use during my flight back to Malta the next day. I was given their contacts in case I needed to get in touch with them and after our formal goodbyes I was taken back to the hotel. Arrangements were made for the next day as they were to collect me to take me to the airport for my flight.

The rest of the day was pretty much a relaxing one as I spent most of the time in my room watching TV, chatting on Skype and browsing the net. Did I mention WIFI in the room is great? I tried the funny cap on but couldn't figure out how I was to wear this as it seemed to cause a little discomfort and at that point decided that the cap wasn't a great idea and perhaps its design could be better. Took my medicine throughout the day and at around 5pm went down for lunch/dinner. Today I tried the fillet of beef again anther nice dish.

I decided to not go out at all that day as it was drizzling and the thought of getting my head wet did not encourage me at all. Even the fact that I could not wear a cap to go out stopped me a bit.

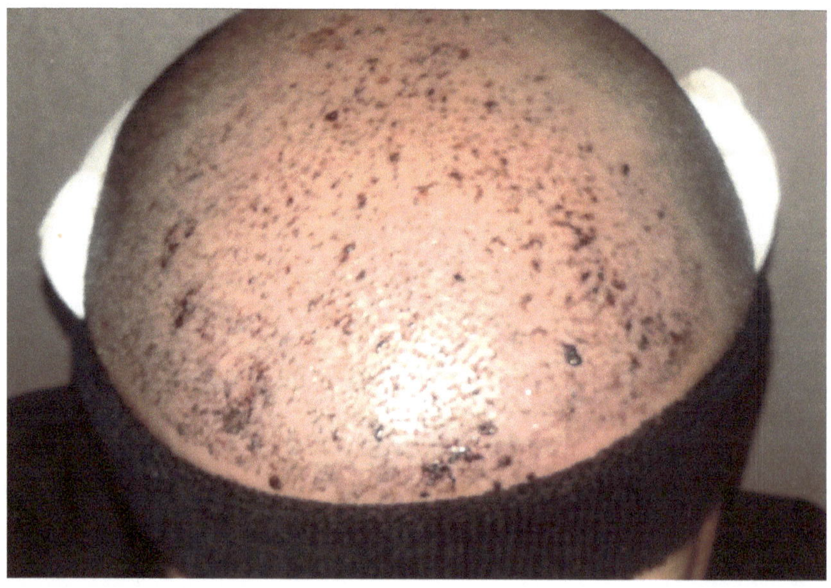

The redness was apparent and there is not much to do about this only time will ease it out and those who would have no idea of what I had done or those who have never seen anyone in this condition before, would be quite shocked to see a man with funny things looking like anything but hair stuck on his slightly red swollen egg head, wearing a bandage under a headband that made me look like a beaten up version of Karate Kid. So it was back to spending some time with my girlfriend on Skype.

DAY 4
12TH APRIL

This morning I woke up at 6am and I must admit that the night was slept well with no sensation of pain or anything that could have disturbed me. I was proud of myself because for the second night running, I had easily managed to maintain my entire sleep in a strict face position throughout the night. I noticed some blood on the special cover placed over the pillow, this was expected but surprisingly not as much as expected.

This day was was also the day I would be catching my flight back home, so before showering I packed some of my bag, then showered and packed the rest, leaving just a few things out but always ready to pack them and go within a minute. I went down for my last breakfast in that restaurant, for the time being, and soon after went up to my room to completely pack and make sure I had left nothing behind. I had time to sit down and watch some news on CNN.

I tried on the hat again and surprisingly the sensation was better than it had felt the previous evening but I still was hesitant to wearing it at that point and pondered on how I would be received by other travelers at the airport if I were to travel without it. I was not embarrassed about what I looked like so thought it would not bother me if other people were looking at me pondering on what I had done to my poor head and decided to proceed to the airport without it.

Adnan was to come and collect me at around 9am, so at 9am I went down to the lobby and as always he was right there on time.

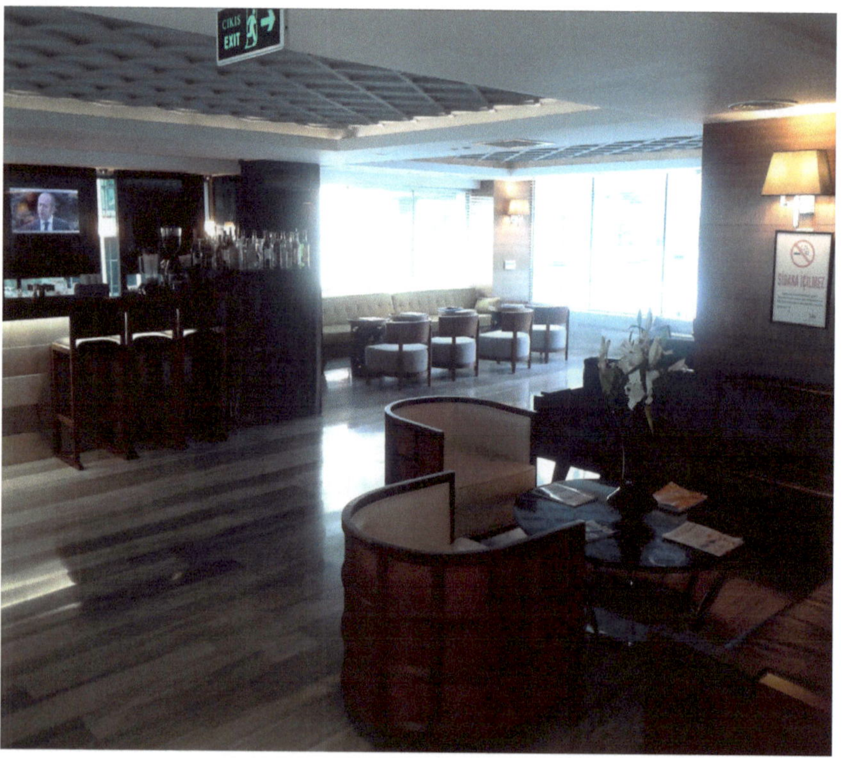

After a quick Turkish tea and a couple of photos together we proceeded to checkout from the hotel and got on the car waiting to take me back to the airport. Adnan accompanied me there, which is why this service was excellent from beginning to end. I still was not wearing my cap once I arrived at the airport and decided not to wear it to see the reactions of the people there. After saying bye to Adnan and Sherat our chauffeur, I made my way to the departure lounge of the airport not wearing any cap. I could see people looking at me and I was wondering to myself if they were perceiving me the way I was perceiving myself, which was as a guy with a swollen red head, that was covered with blood dried spots on top, wearing a sweatband with the Doctor's name and a white slightly blood stained bandage at the back under the sweatband. I noticed that balding men were taking lots of interest in me and would be taking long glimpses of me when they thought I was not noticing, turning their sights as soon as I would look their way. Men with hair just stared at me, apparently with a complex expression, perhaps either wondering what was it I had or thanking their lucky stars that it's not them or probably just trying to understand the situation. Together with these, there were quite a few people who gave me filthy looks, as if I was an outcast or as if I seemed to have some sort of funny disease. Completely bald men looked at me quite evilly as if they wanted to tell me that they would never stoop so low or perhaps because they couldn't have it done themselves maybe because of a poor donor area. Some women seemed indifferent, others not so, especially those with the husbands with a full set of hair who just stared with no apparent sign of any sort of emotion. Some people frowned a little, these must have been the type that could not bear to see the sight of anything macabre or blood. I don't blame the latter, this is how I probably would have reacted had I seen the same thing on someone else. Even the slightest thought of blood makes my legs wobbly like jelly and my head spin like the roulette.

I pushed it a bit more and checked in and proceeded to the long queue for the passport control and hand luggage X-ray machines. A Maltese man recognised me and asked me what happened so I told him the truth, which was that I had come to Turkey to have a Hair transplant, which I had the previous evening. He congratulated me and wished me good luck. The queue leading to the final passport control and security check was the most annoying part of this experience as there is many lanes in a two way position so I had a long line of people looking at me from one end and another from the other end and each. As soon as I passed the X-ray machine and final security check point I decided that it was time to wear the cap not because I was embarrassed or felt bullied by those looking at me strangely but mainly because I didn't want to disgust the people boarding the same plane with me. The cap hid the fact completely and although it looked kind of weird on my head, or should I say stupid, it changed people's attitude completely and people were either not noticing me and those that did, did not seem to bother about what I was wearing. I boarded the plane and kept the cap throughout the whole flight and this was not at all uncomfortable.

On the plane I met an old school friend of mine whom I had not seen for quite some time and he wondered what had brought me to Istanbul obviously not noting anything beneath the hat. Seeing that his hair was also residing, it was no trouble being honest with him and explained to him what I had done. I would have told him the truth anyway. He was enthusiastic about it and confessed that he was looking into it himself. I had some time to explain the procedure briefly before the plane took off and he was hooked. Unfortunately he was sitting in a different section so our short encounter ended up with an appointment to contact each other on FB so that I can meet him and discuss all the details. The flight back home was comfortable and hassle free and we reached our destination on good time. Passing through security check and customs was easier that I was expecting it to be, so this was nice and simple and I had no problems passing through with the medications. My girlfriend was waiting outside, eager to see me and eager to get a glimpse of the results of the op. I too was eager to show her but decided that the airport was not the right place and waited until we arrived home.

As soon as we reached home and were indoors I was keen to show her my transplant but was hesitant that most probably she would dislike the current swollen and redness look, so I asked her if she would like to see the transplant. Of course she did, so I took of the cap and everything was very fine. The only thing that made the thing look worse than it actually was, was the slightly blood stained bandage under the headband, but I told her that the doctor said that this was normal during the first couple or so days. The rest of the day was spent at home, relaxing and taking the medications as prescribed and preparing the things needed for when I sleep at night. I also had to remove the bandage and treat my head with the special cream and shampoo provided but I thought of preparing some additional things.

Feeling a little uncomfortable going out, not because I was shy or not feeling well enough to do so but mainly because I wanted to avoid exposing my head to any dust or sun, I asked my girlfriend to go and purchase some baby changing sheets from the pharmacy and some gauze bandages. I wanted these in case I needed it for under the head band, which I had to keep on for yet another day after cleansing my head as instructed the previous day. I knew there was no need for the bandage, but still wanted to place some gauze under the headband at the back of my head as I was thinking about the worse possible scenario i.e. should my head bleed at night and the headband get stuck directly to the raw skin. The supplies were easily and cheaply available at my local pharmacy, so within a few minutes my girlfriend came back with supplies from the pharmacy that is located just around the corner from where we live. It was now time to apply the cleansing treatment myself for the first time.

First I took off the sweatband but left the bandage at the back of my head since this adhered to my skin due to the dried blood and I did not have the courage to pull it off as I was worried that I may open up any wound and blood would start flowing again. But I had a plan that worked very nicely indeed. When I removed the headband I applied the 1st part foam lotion to the top of my scalp where the new hair was implanted and left the foam to work its magic for 30 minutes as instructed. Once the 30mins were up, then I had to rinse the foam off gently with lukewarm water and apply the second process, shampooing and cleansing part of the whole head. I still had the bandage adhered to the back of my head, so I ran my head under a gentle stream of lukewarm water firstly to rinse off the foam as instructed but also to wet the bandage so that it can come off easily without any addition force from my behalf. The bandage came off quite easily as I gently pulled it with minimal pain and with no signs of any blood flowing down. As soon as the bandage was off I applied the second part of the cleansing treatment using the special shampoo. Once this was applied I rinsed the shampoo off again with lukewarm water and dried my head as instructed, patting it gently all around using paper towels.

Once the cleansing process was over, I showered the rest of my body making sure no water from the shower hits any part of my head. I was very curious to what I would see at the back of my head so as once as I had finished and dried myself I got a glimpse of the sight from a hand held mirror pointing at the mirror on the wall. I was quite impressed at the healing process at the back of my headband everything looked quite fine indeed.

Since I decided to document this in full and make this a photographic journey commencing from the day of the surgery, I took my first set of photos. I will continue to do this for the next 12months on a weekly basis, to see for myself how the process is undergoing and to show others who want this information. It will provide a honest and a real evaluation of the final results of the operation. After taking my first set of photos, I then reapplied a small narrow piece of the gauze bandage not much wider than the headband strip, under where the sweatband would be resting against the rear of my head as I didn't want the sweatband to adhere to my raw but healing skin at that point and applied the sweatband making the bandage now completely invisible. The rest of the day was spent simply watching TV and surfing on the net.

When it came to bedtime, I covered the pillow with the baby changing towels and slept as I had done the previous two nights, face up. I was wondering what this towel would be looking like in the morning, my thoughts were that it would be soaked in blood since I now had no bandage to absorb any blood that may come out during the night. Since I was applying pressure to the back of my head against the pillow, I was expecting the worst but there was only one way to find out and morning will tell.

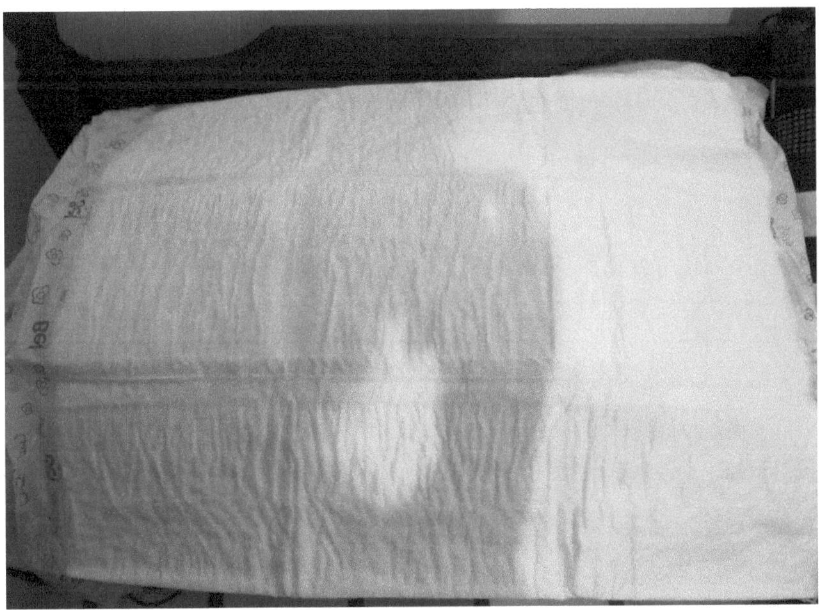

DAY 5
13TH APRIL

This morning I woke up at around 7am after yet another good night's sleep in which I didn't twist or turn in bed at all, waking up face up just like in the last past days. I am really surprised at myself but I am guessing that the subconscious and often conscious thought lingering at the back of my mind about taking care of these implants, due to the long process of the op, is keeping me from doing so, at least for now.

As now is the case, the first thing I did was to take a look at the baby changing protective sheet placed on the pillow to see signs of blood. Surprisingly enough there was none except for some minor traces of faded blood where the headband was. The blood though wasn't fresh blood from the wound that flowed during the night but blood that passed through the previous bandage from the previous night, that was soaked in by the sweatband and which must have transferred to the protective sheet because I had sweated slightly during the night due to feeling hot with our thick warm quilt.

I looked in the mirror to take a look at my head and all was looking fairly good. I am very happy with the initial progress so far, no blood from the back and the top seems to be healing nicely.

Today is my final day with the head band, so I will finally disown the karate kid look and believe me it will be a relieve to be without it tomorrow! I am planning to go out today but will be wearing my cap as the top of my head is still a quite red and sore looking but I am in no pain at all and to be quite honest very comfortable at the moment. I took my morning pill after breakfast and shortly after went out to have lunch outside with my girlfriend and took the second course of pills after lunch. As soon as I returned home after a Sunday drive around the countryside, I began the cleansing process, so I removed the headband, an easy task, and I removed the narrow gauze strip I had placed under the headband in order to prevent the headband from sticking to my head should I have opened any wound during the night. However since I did not bleed the gauze just came off easily and no blood was apparent on the gauze, "A very good sign" , I thought to myself, because I hate the sight of blood. I went through the cleansing process as the previous day, taking care of patting the foam gently over the implants, rinsing well under a gentle stream of lukewarm water and applying the shampoo over the whole of my head and rinsing it off again.

The whole process takes about 40-45mins, 30mins of which can be spent in front of the computer or TV, or reading a book waiting for the foam to soak into the scalp and do its magic. After rinsing and paper towel drying my head I took my daily photos that I have posted in the daily photo log in the member's area free with this book.

I carried on the rest of the evening relaxing, as anyone should do on a Sunday evening, until it was time to sleep. Preparing to sleep was now a simple routine of placing the protective cover over the pillow and laying my head to sleep face up. I can't remember falling asleep but it must have been instant.

DAY 6
14TH APRIL

This was the 6th day from my life changing experience and I woke up early morning after another good night's sleep. As I have done for the past few days, the moment I woke up I checked to see if there was any blood on the protective cover placed on the pillow. To my delight there was not even a single drop or a sign of it. I was still wearing the headband and a narrow strip of gauze bandage behind the headband just in case there is blood in order to avoid the headband sticking to my skin should the wounds, especially the injection wounds, start bleeding.

The gauze would be much easier to remove than the headband if that was the case. That day the headband finally came off and this was the first thing I did after breakfast and before my shower. I was extremely happy that the headband came off easily as expected and the gauze did too, with no signs of blood and no adhesion to the skin. The healing process was going very well.

For the past few days I have been doing the cleaning process early afternoon, but that day I decided to get it done between 11am and noon, so that the next day I can do it at around 10am and from the days that followed will be able to fit in in my usual daily routine at 9am. As planned I cleansed my head using the usual process at around 11:30am and then continued to shower the rest of my body. Wearing and taking off tops and t-shirts has now become easier than the first couple of days and I have been doing this very carefully as to not touch any of the affected areas. I spent an early afternoon indoors doing some work online. After sometime at my desk working, I started to get a bit bored, feeling a little contained because I had not stepped foot outside for the past few days. So I decided to take a drive and drove myself, for the first time in a week, to my mother's place, to show her the result. So far the only persons to have seen me like this post op were the surgeons, the people in the hotel in Istanbul, the people at the airport and my girlfriend. My mother had not seen me yet.

When I arrived at her home and showed her the results so far, to my surprise, she was sincerely delighted and honestly told me it looks great. For the first time she confessed that she preferred me with hair than with a bald look and she was looking forward to seeing more of it soon. Initially I hadn't told my mother that I was planning to do the op until a week prior to me leaving but now I knew that she would have been supportive and positive about it had I mentioned it to her before. People never cease to surprise me! Upon returning home, I spent the rest of the day writing my journal, the one you are reading in this book.

That night was to be the first night that I would be sleeping without any headband and no bandage what so ever, however I decided and planned to place the protective cover over the pillow just in case. The daily medications as prescribed did not give me any unwanted or undesired side effects, in any way, that was a positive sign and a great relief. At that point I was still a little worried that whilst sleeping I may hit my head, where the implants have been implanted, against the headboard so was very cautious to place the pillow a little further down to try and avoid this from happening as much as possible. My girlfriend was very supportive when I had less hair, but I think she secretly likes the new look, perhaps it reminded her of my younger me?

DAY 7
15TH APRIL

This day was the last day to be reporting about my progress in this book, especially since things have become quite repetitive and the processes are now turning into routines. I did have another good night's rest the previous night although the donor area was itching due to the healing process. However despite this itchiness, that I have been able to resists, I am happy to report that there was no sign of blood on any part of the protective sheet. I guess the healing process from the donor area is the way it should be. It felt a little bit scabby at the back but it was a real relief to sleep without the sweatband for the first time since the operation. I was hoping that things will be good enough to be able to go out not wearing any sort of cap in the days that followed. I looked in the mirror and noticed that the swelling effect was gradually fading and things are looked quite good on top too. If you are wondering what the top feels like, then take a wire brush, the type with hard bristles and pat your hand over the tips of the bristles. This is what the implants feel like, during the first few weeks of a transplant, when you pat them gently. Eventually after time they become normal and unnoticeable just like real hair.

I made it a point to commence the cleansing process earlier than the day before at around 10:00am, right after taking my breakfast and first morning pill. The cleansing process was as usual, started with applying the foam on the implanted area and leaving it absorb for 30mins, then rinsed the area with lukewarm water and after washed the entire scalp with the special shampoo provided and rinsed it all off again, paper towel dried the head afterwards. The process is very simple and easily fits into a daily routine. Afterwards I showered and took some photos which you can see in the photo section. Being the last day to be reporting, I dedicated time to ensure all the details were as correct as could be and I remember thinking to myself that the idea of having this book written was a very good one and feeling glad that I have dedicated a lot of time to do so in the hope that it will be very helpful to others in the future.

I spent most of the day indoors, working on the book and photos I had so far. I never imagined that I would be dedicating so much time to this project but the more I wrote the more I felt committed to provide a complete source of information for those needing it. Initially, the idea was to have this information freely available to everyone, but had second thoughts during those first few days as I felt that this information should only be available to those who require it. I felt that it was only fair that those really interested should have access to my personal experience and photos.

I have been going out since my operation almost on a daily basis after the first couple of days, and today I went out for a brief walk around the area I live in. It is good to have some fresh air and exercise a little. I wear the cap as my head is still not that presentable for public viewing at the moment. I get sympathy pains myself whenever I see someone who has any sort of medical condition and would not like to do that to anyone else. Also since most people did not know what I had done, the implanted area and the donor area may have appeared to be some sort of funny disease or contagious medical condition and I didn't want people to think things of the sort. I would prefer they know the truth, but if people don't know you they will never ask you, hence will only most probably assume.

The cap the clinic provided looked a little silly on me. I felt like a wet India Jones wearing it. But it was comfortable and although I tried other caps, none were as comfortable at it. I was also afraid that other types of caps may interfere in the healing process so I preferred looking silly than compromising the operation or extending the healing process. A few friends around the area knew that I had gone ahead and had a hair transplant operation and because the village I live in is small, word spread like wildfire in a short period, which was good because I didn't have to invent excuses and soon after I was able to go out wearing no cap at all.

From my introduction, you know that I work in show business so that day I was happy when I felt good enough to perform my usual weekly rehearsals without any problems what so ever. I was not expecting to be back at rehearsals a few days after the op but I was quite happy I did. However I must say that I left my input as minimal as possible, so that I did not sweat at all, or overdo it with any type of physical strain or apply any pressure on my body especially my head at that point. The people working around me knew that I had done a transplant so showing it to them and spending time with them was no issue at all. We mostly worked on things they would be doing at that point. After rehearsals I went home, ate, took all my medications and continued logging my day, which is what you are reading right now.

That day I managed to finish one set of pills, the little white ones. The following day, I would have finished off another set and by the next day I would have complete the whole medication. I am extremely happy that I didn't take the pain killers provided since

I did not need them at all which I consider to be excellent. At 11:30pm I set to log my very last report in this book. The past seven days have been a good experience without any hitches and from that perspective I felt content to have risked going to Istanbul. Had I the information in this book available I wouldn't have had a second thought of going before I actually geared up enough courage to go through it. The 7 days of reporting my progress, which was excellent, was also a great exercise in understanding the whole process, making sure I was doing everything correct and personally it also helped me.

I was happy that I didn't need to report any disadvantages, or regrets and believe me there weren't. It was at that point that I decided to go a step further and provide a good conclusion for this book, one that was to be written within a week of this last day.

CONCLUSION
(WRITTEN ON THE 15TH DAY AFTER THE OPERATION)
22ND APRIL

I am wrote this conclusion exactly a week after the very last day of reporting all my seven day experience in this book. My experience was not as bad as I had imagined it would have been during the time I was waiting for the day to come. As a matter of fact it was a very smooth experience with minimal effect on me up to this day, and as can be seen in the photo I have very good progress.

During the week that passed, I started entering my normal daily routines. I was also going out in the evenings without any sort of cap. In the day time I chose to wear a cap only to protect my scalp from the sun. However I wasn't wearing the silly had given to me after the operation, by then I was wearing a normal baseball cap, measured to its full extension so that I could easily put on and take off without disrupting the implants in any way.

As warned and as I read, I had lost a few of the implants but this was a normal process. It is because a small percentage of the roots extracted may not have lived during the transplant process. Unfortunately there is no way of knowing if or any of the roots have died until after being implanted and waiting for a few weeks or so. However this was so minimal that it did not affect the appearance or progress in any way.

I also had time to re-read the book and am amazed at the amount of details I have provided is so informative in such a personal detailed account. I am still not able to find such information collected in one place easily accessible and readable up to this day.

Based on my experience, I wouldn't discourage anyone considering this procedure. Having it done in Turkey was also a good choice. It was cheaper than having it done elsewhere, the procedure was top class and the after care is top notch. Kaan kept in touch with me quite a few times since the operation and that made me feel very comfortable.

However I still had to wait at least another seven months to see some better results. There was a whole process I had to endure in order to see the result. I was looking forward to seeing the roots sprout with the baby hair, was not looking forward to seeing those baby hairs fall again, but was really excited about the new hairs after the baby hairs have fallen to start growing. These were the hairs that were meant to last.

It took me over two weeks to write and finish off the note for this book and it will take me more time to make them readable plus another 52 weeks to document the weekly photos.

Those photos will be in the next and final chapter.

THE FINAL CHAPTER
9TH APRIL THE FOLLOWING YEAR

It's been exactly 1 year to date since I had my hair transplant operation in Turkey. During the past months, Kaan continued to keep in contact with me. The progress was astonishing and the process was as smooth as it could have gone. I am a happier man now, although I spend almost 45mins to do my hair. It's amazing what a difference a little bit of hair can do to a man who has lost it at an early stage in their life. I feel more confident about my appearance and being in show business I feel like I bring over a better performance when entertaining audiences as I do not have to think about my hair any more and can focus on what I am doing.

During the past 52 weeks, I went through all the steps I was expecting to go through. Baby hairs started to sprout within the first few weeks. Then I experienced a brief period of hair loss again once these started to fall out,as they are meant to during the process, and be replaced with the hair that is meant to last. The real change started to become more apparent once all the new baby hairs had been replaced and the new hairs started to grow. By that time I was able to comb and style my hair. I also chose to use a certain shampoo, that has proved quite efficient. The shampoo I chose to use, and continue to use is called 'Cystiphane Biorga'. It has no added perfumes, is designed to control hair loss and I have found that it adds volume to my hair. So that pleased me very much. To style my hair I use 'Nivea Styling Cream Gel'. I chose this particular brand and type after much research, looking for a suitable product that contains as little chemicals and perfumes as possible that could affect the natural process of hair.

Looking at all the photos I am adding to this book, it amazing how a little bit of hair can change your appearance. Most importantly it has changed my inner feelings. It has also taught me how to respect other parts of my physical being because even if there may be cures or procedures to cure or regain or fix the parts of your body that bother you, nothing is quite like having a good function natural body. Would I recommend the procedure to anyone?

Take a look at the photos that follow and decide for yourself.

PHOTO LOG

3 Days After The Operation

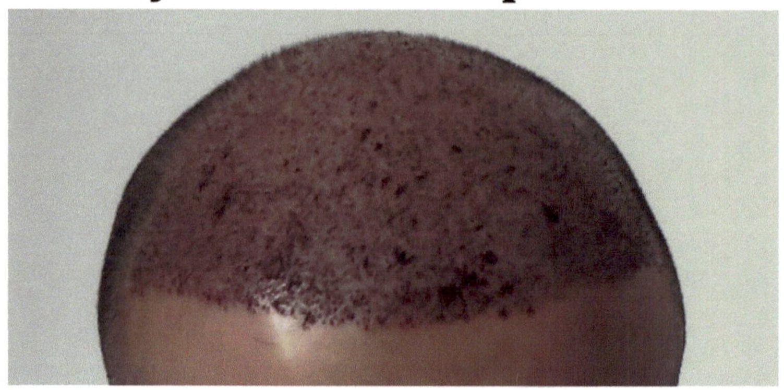

After 1 Week

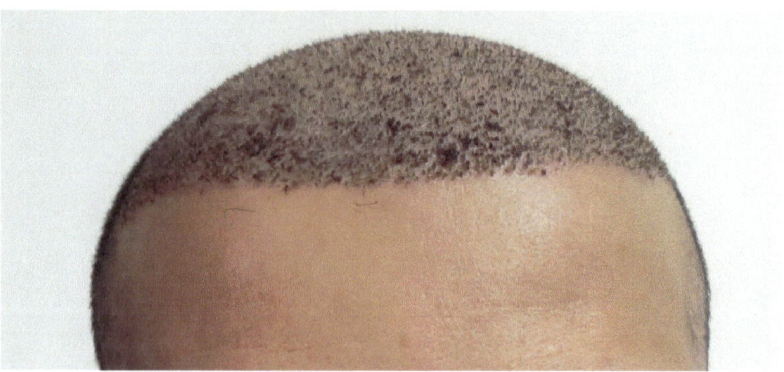

After 2 Weeks

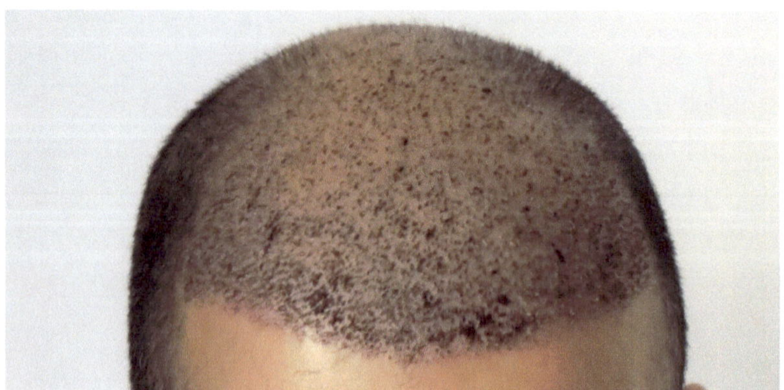

After 3 Weeks

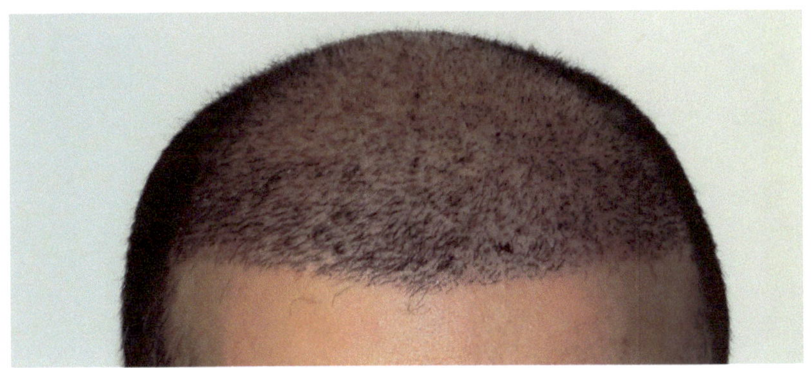

After 4 Weeks

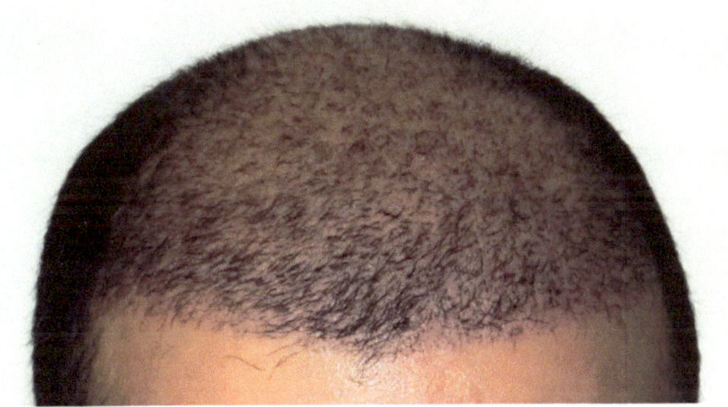

After 5 Weeks

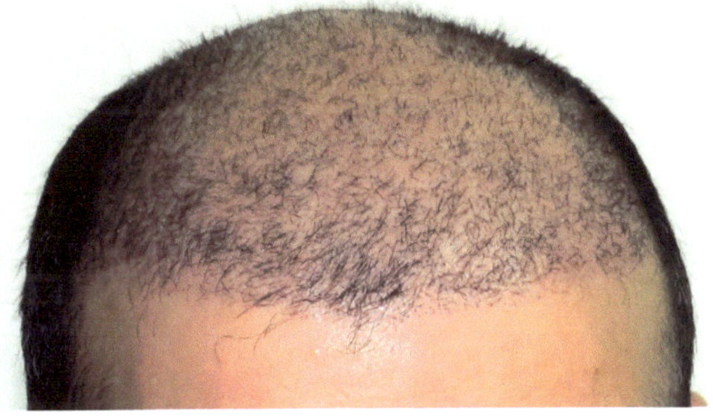

After 6 Weeks

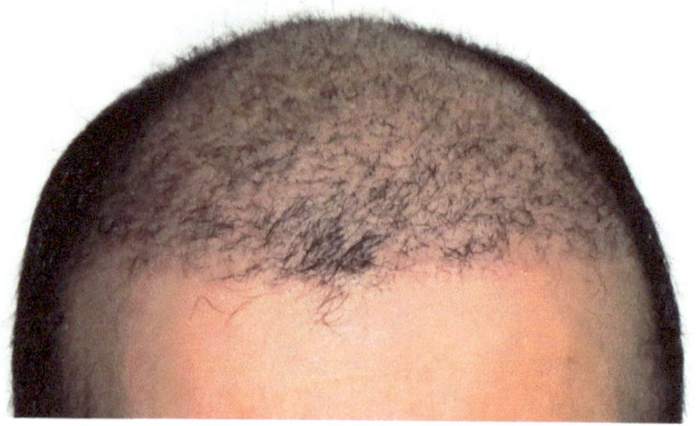

After 7 Weeks

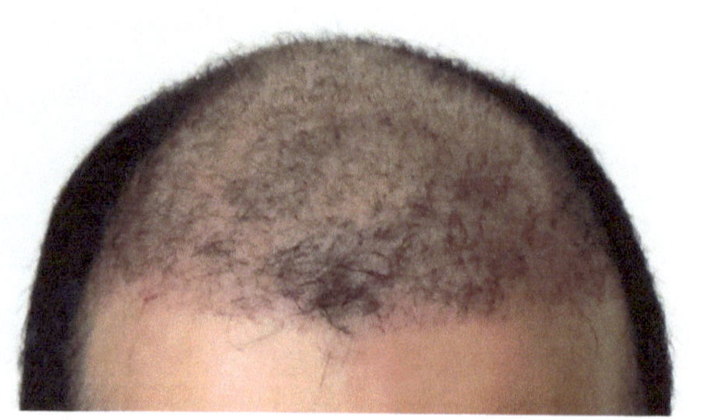

After 8 Weeks

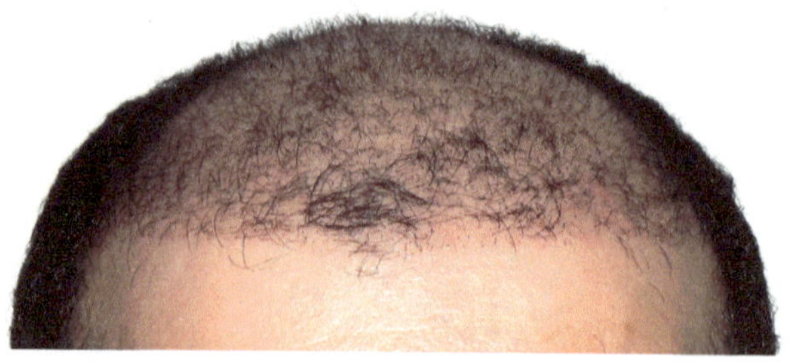

After 9 Weeks

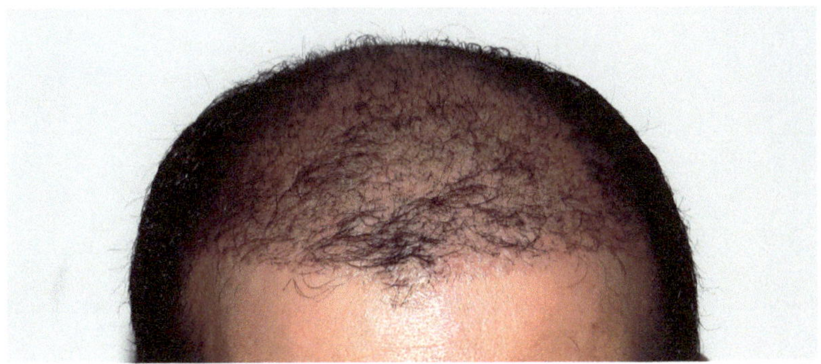

After 10 Weeks

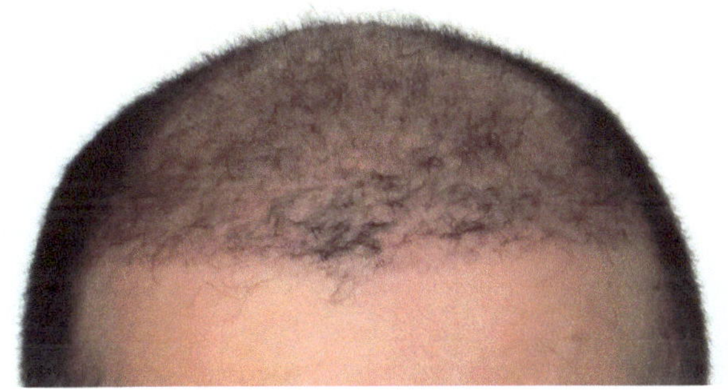

After 11 Weeks

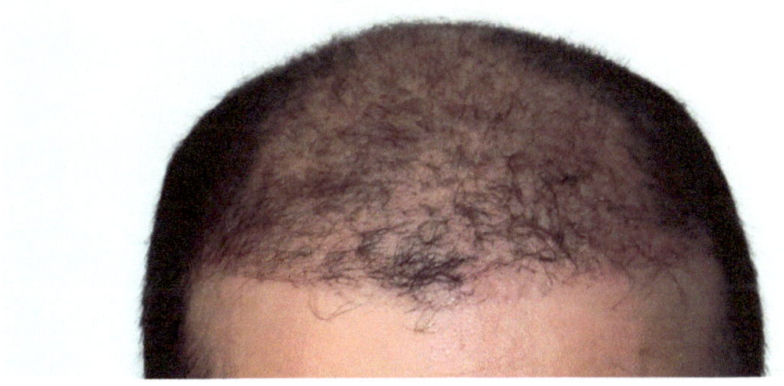

After 12 Weeks

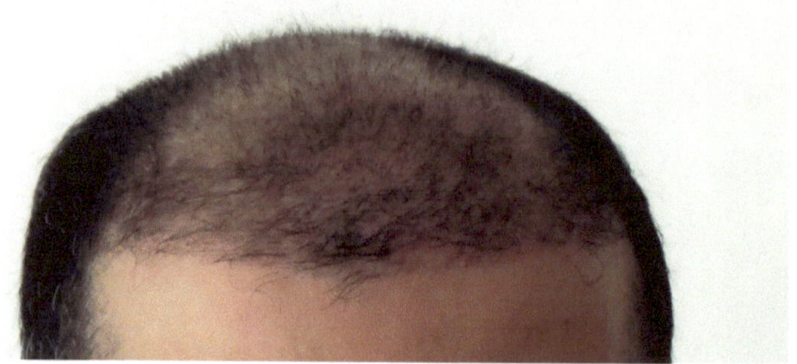

After 13 Weeks

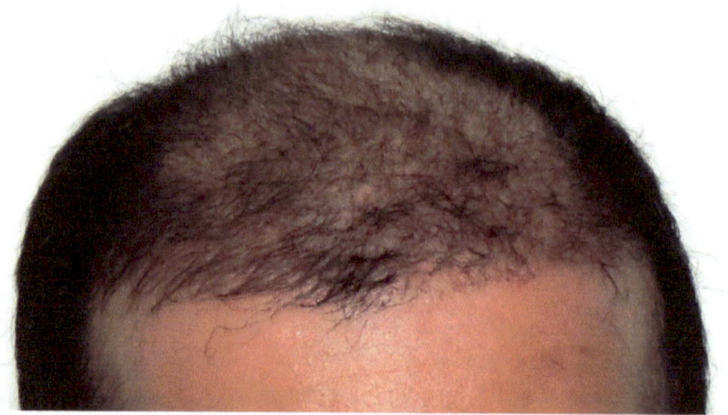

After 14 Weeks

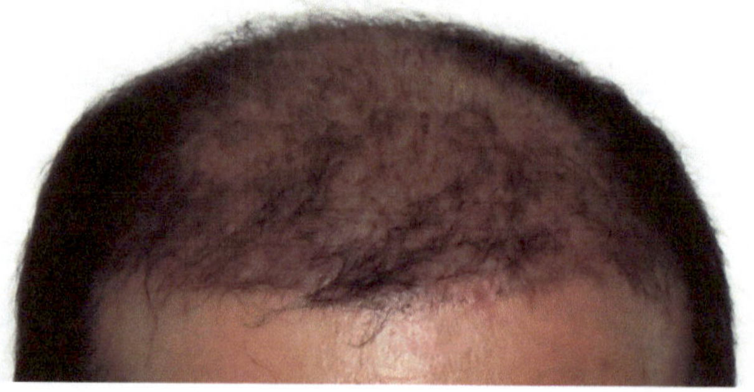

After 15 Weeks

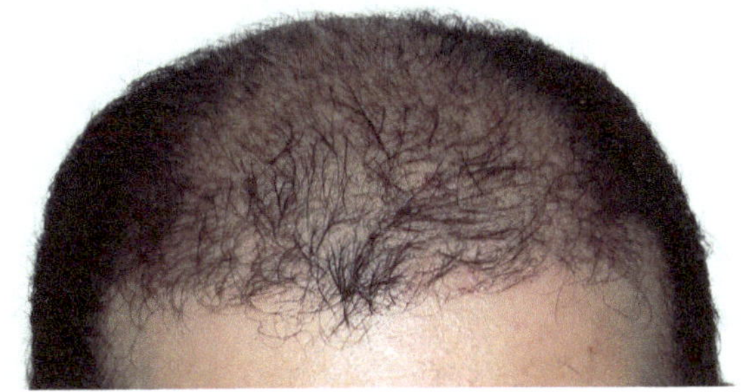

After 16 Weeks

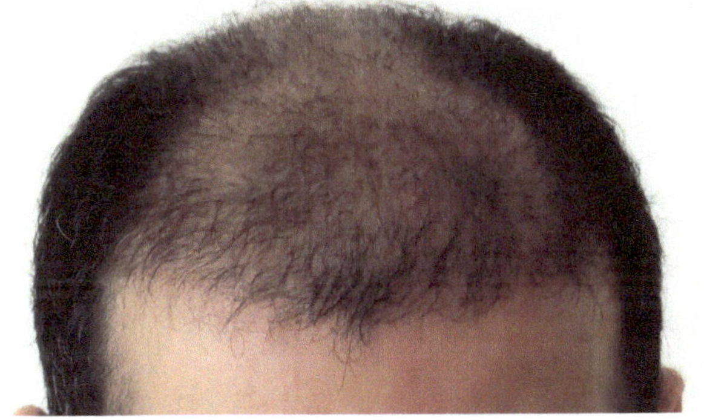

After 17 Weeks

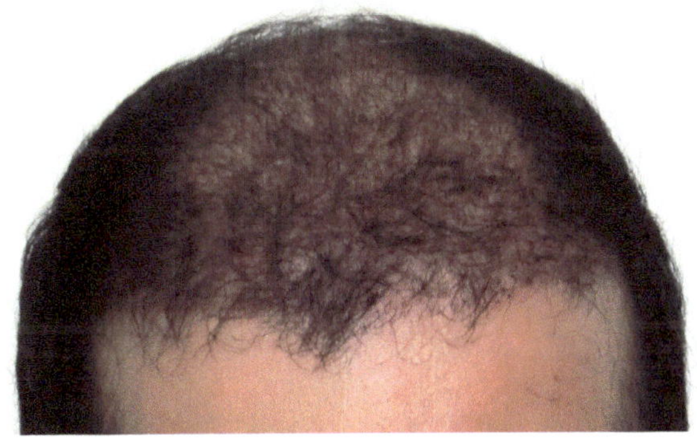

After 18 Weeks

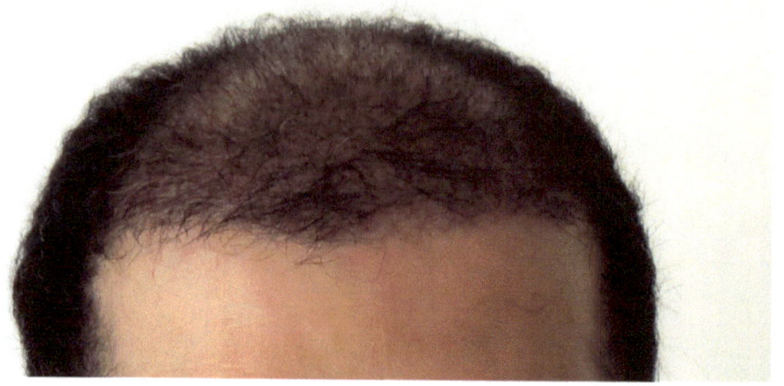

After 19 Weeks

(and my first haircut after the op)

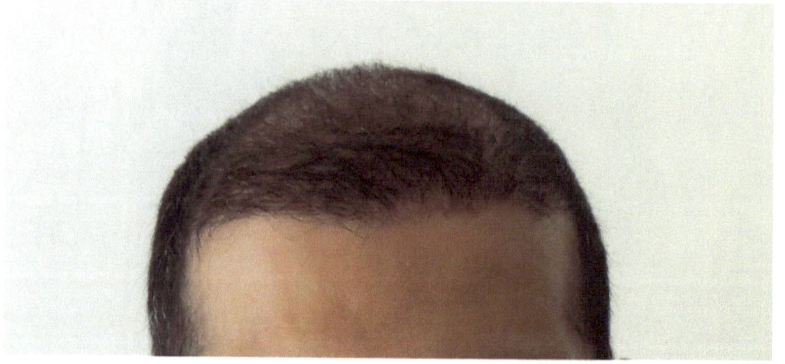

After 20 Weeks

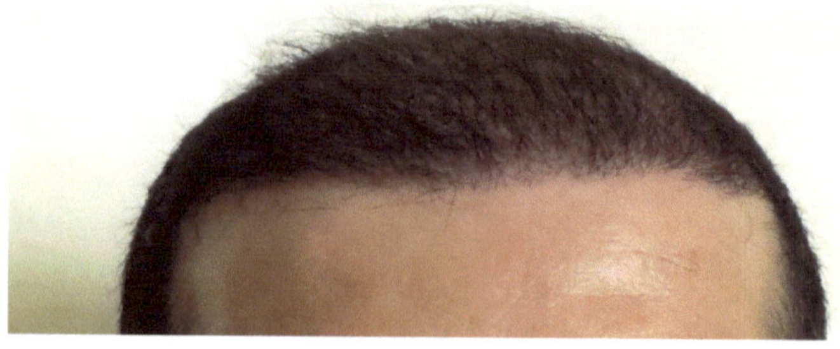

After 21 Weeks

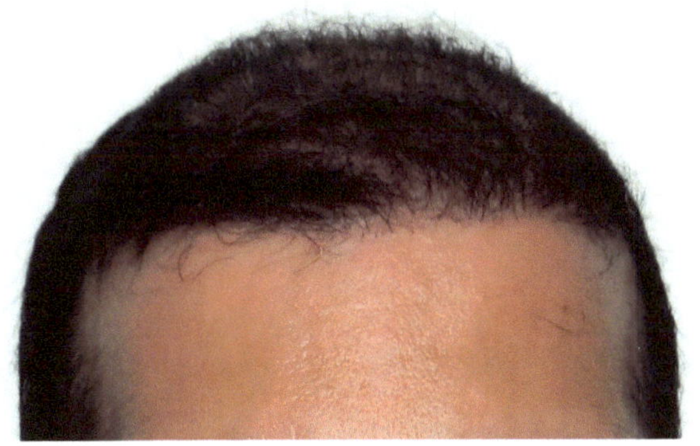

After 22 Weeks

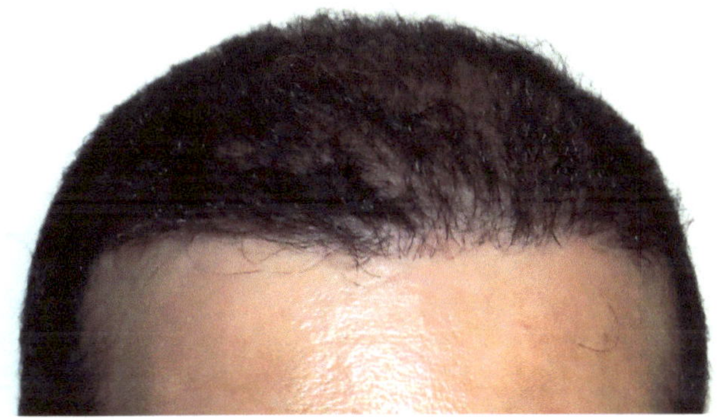

After 23 Weeks

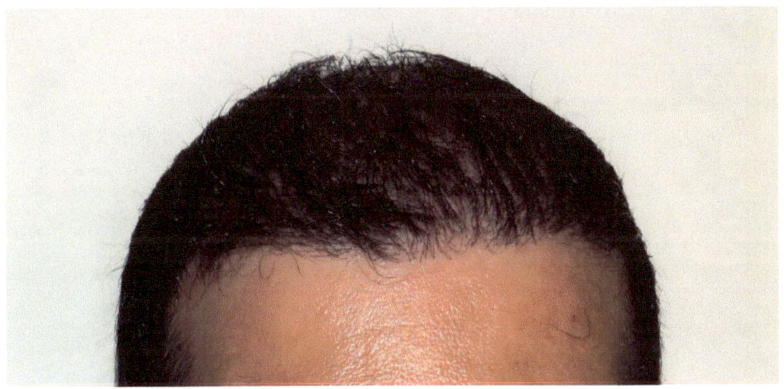

After 24 Weeks

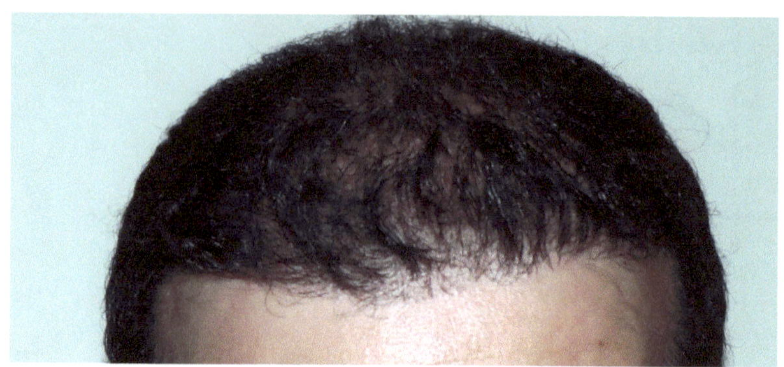

After 25 Weeks

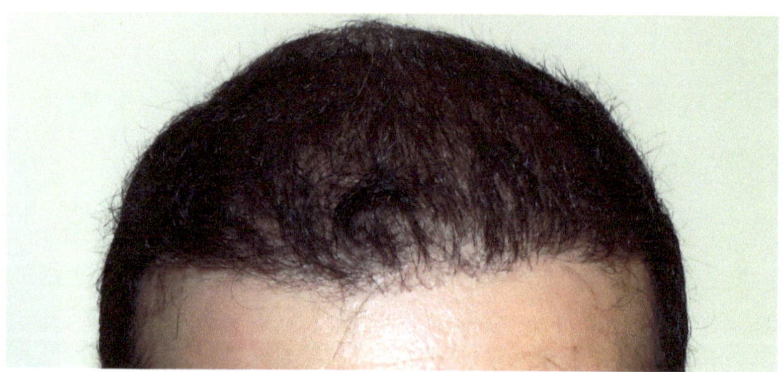

After 26 Weeks

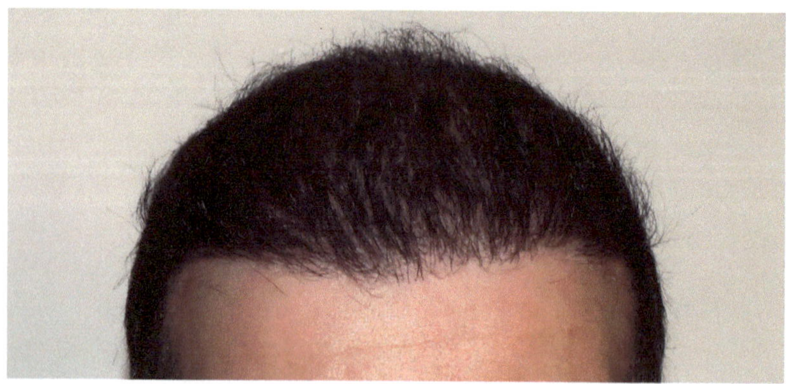

After 27 Weeks

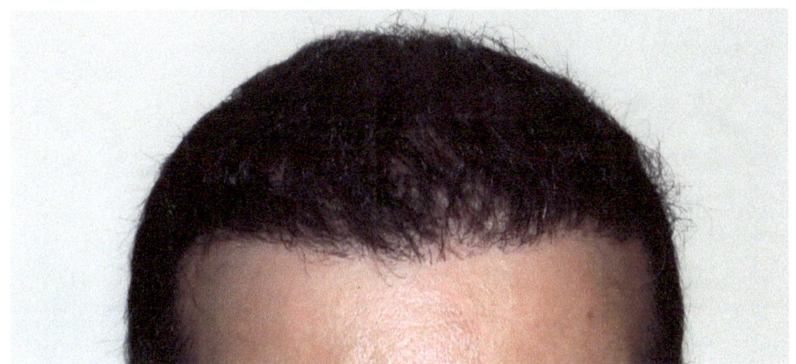

After 28 Weeks

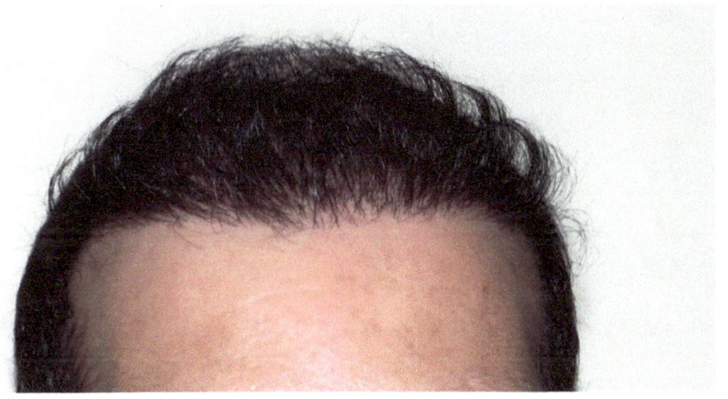

After 29 Weeks

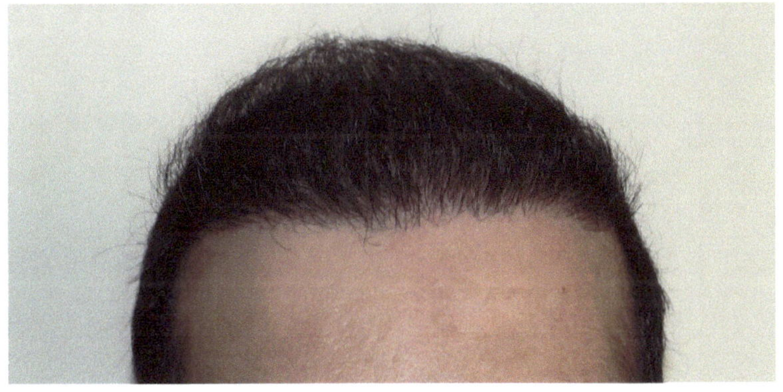

After 30 Weeks

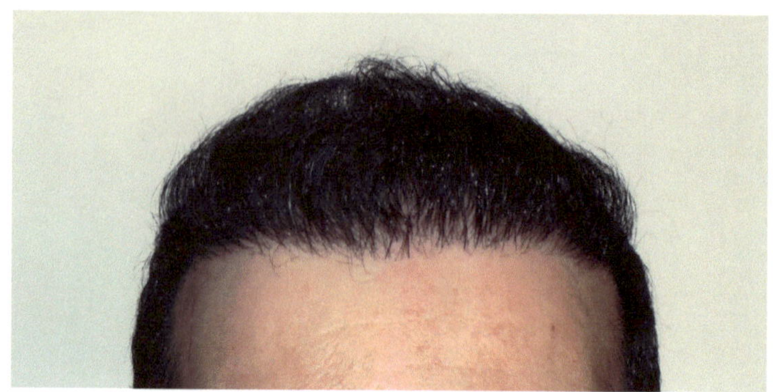

After 31 Weeks

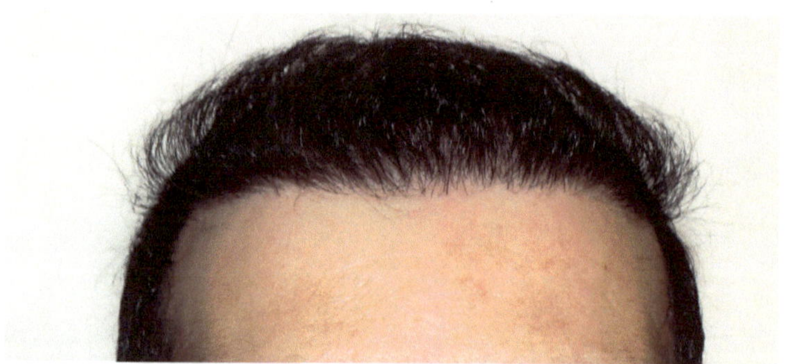

After 32 Weeks

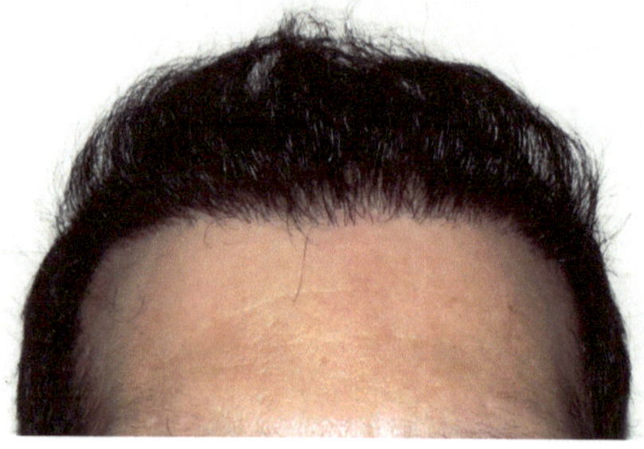

After 33 Weeks

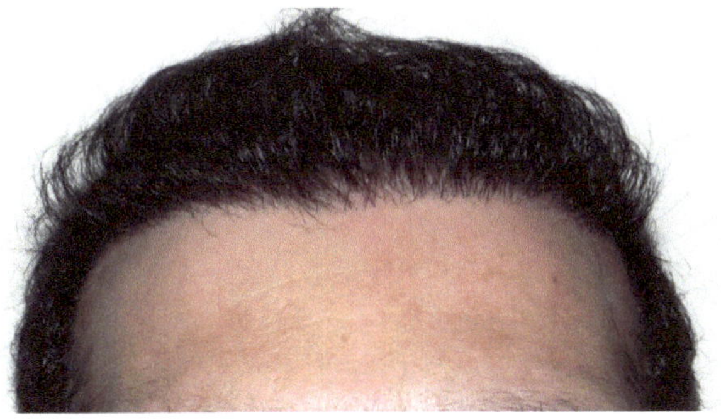

After 34 Weeks

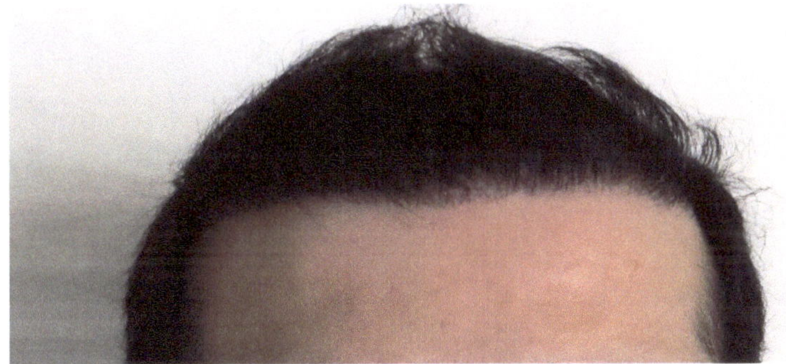

After 35 Weeks

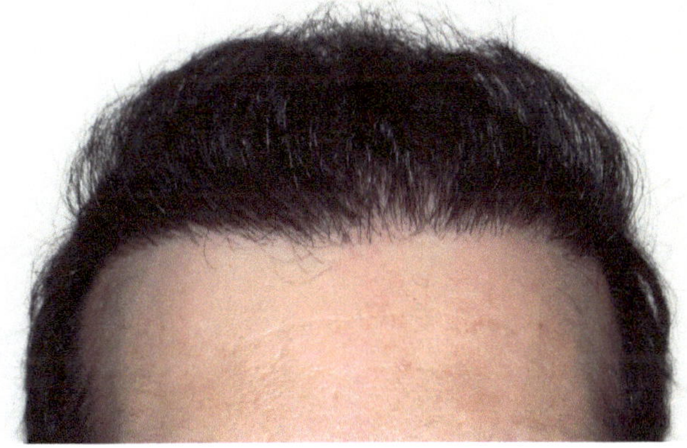

After 36 Weeks

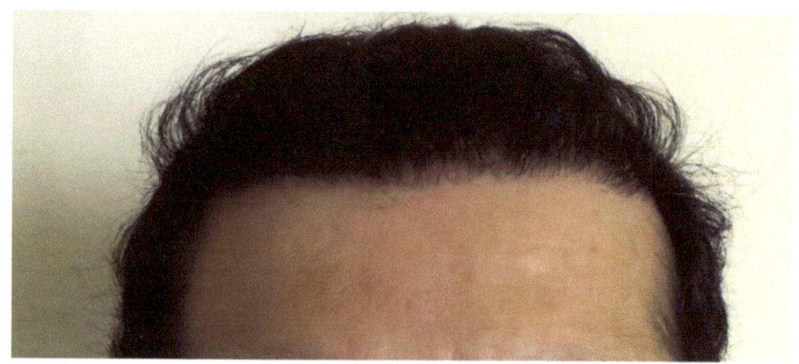

After 37 Weeks

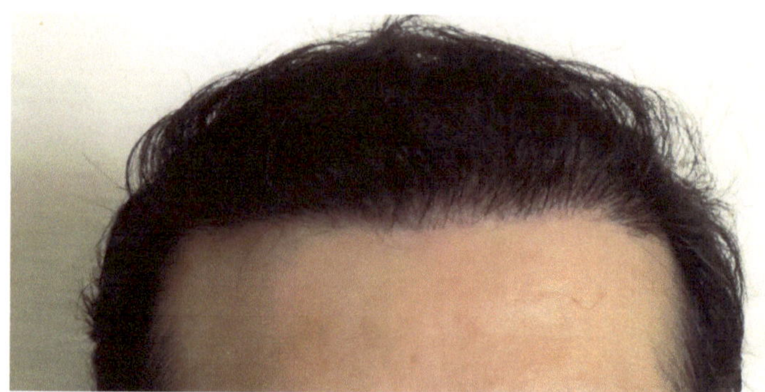

After 38 Weeks

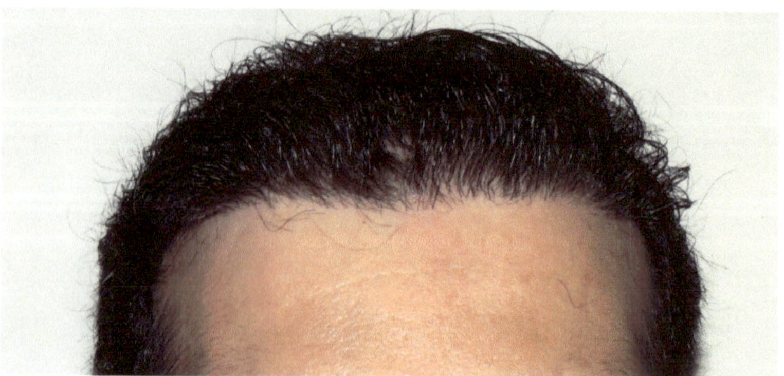

After 39 Weeks

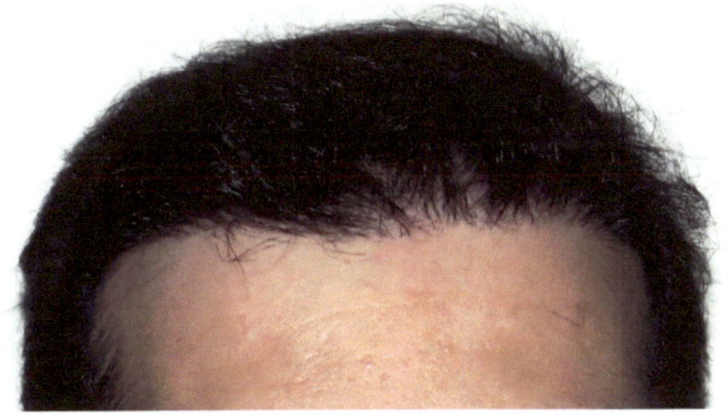

After 40 Weeks

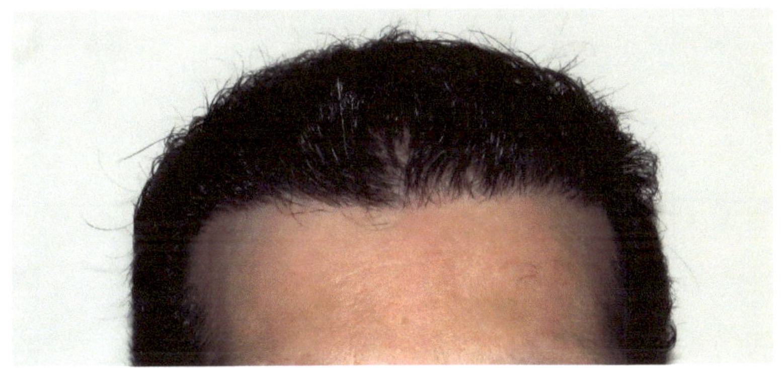

After 41 Weeks

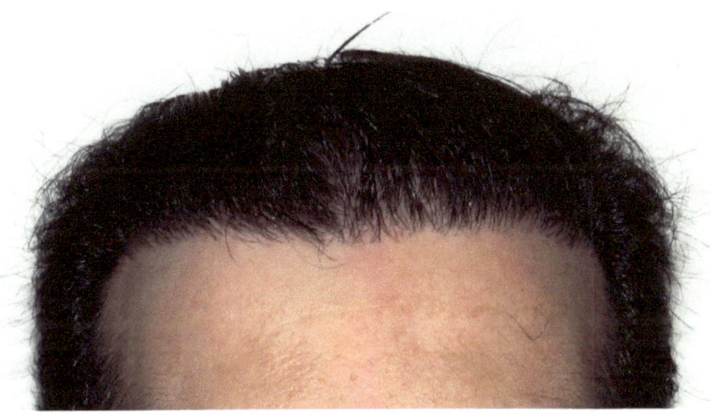

After 42 Weeks

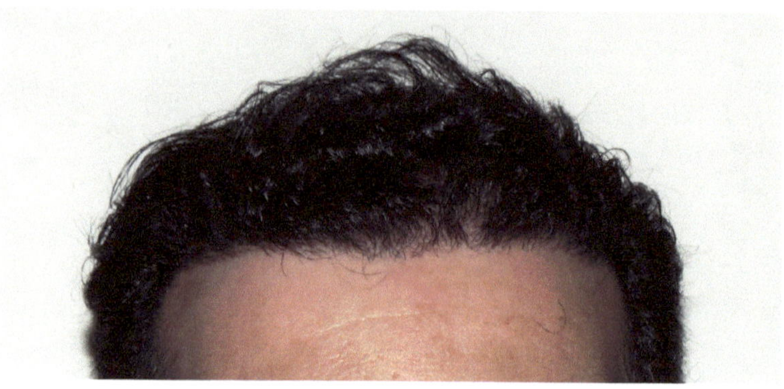

After 43 Weeks

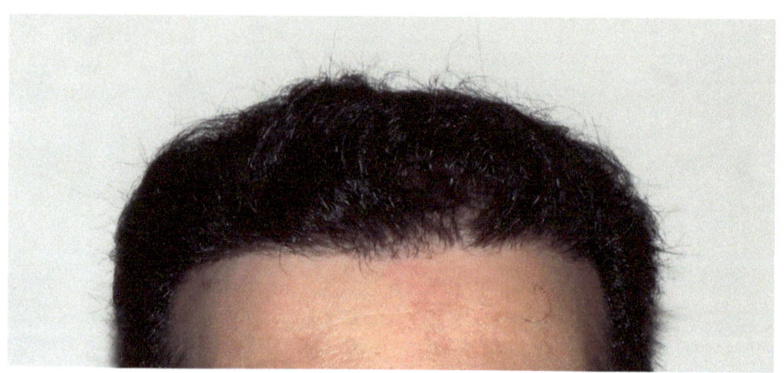

After 44 Weeks

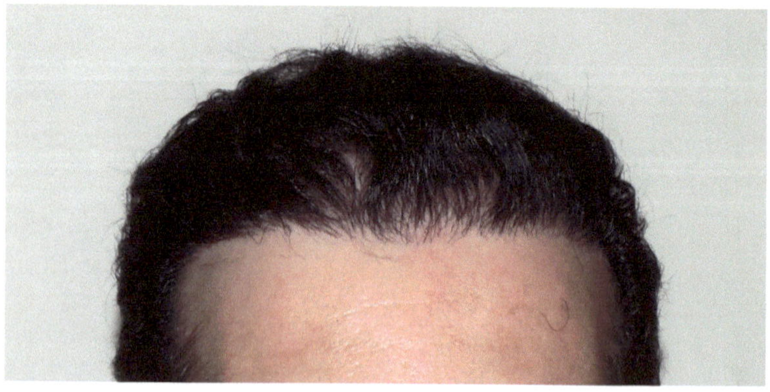

After 45 Weeks

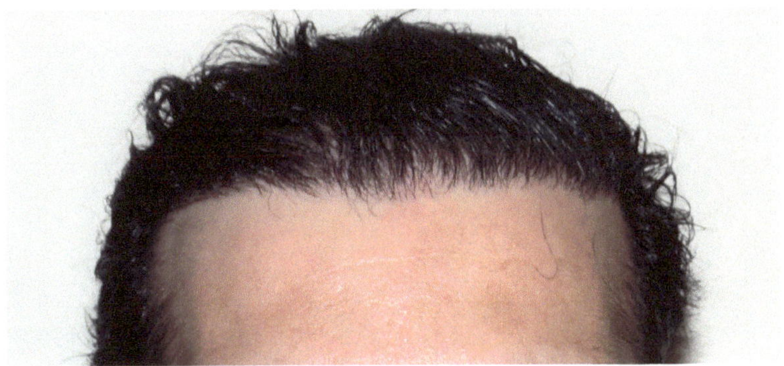

After 46 Weeks

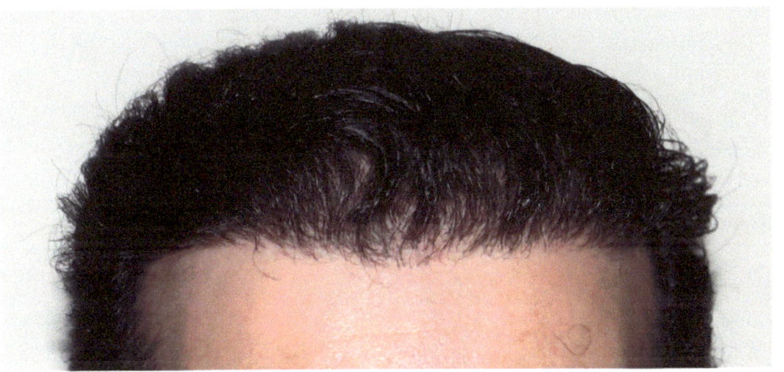

After 47 Weeks

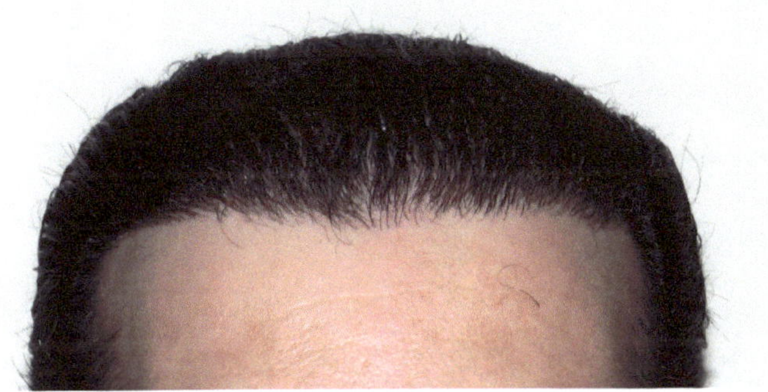

After 48 Weeks

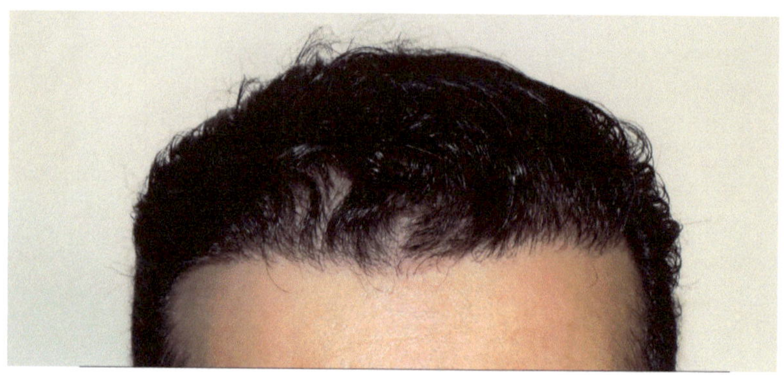

After 49 Weeks

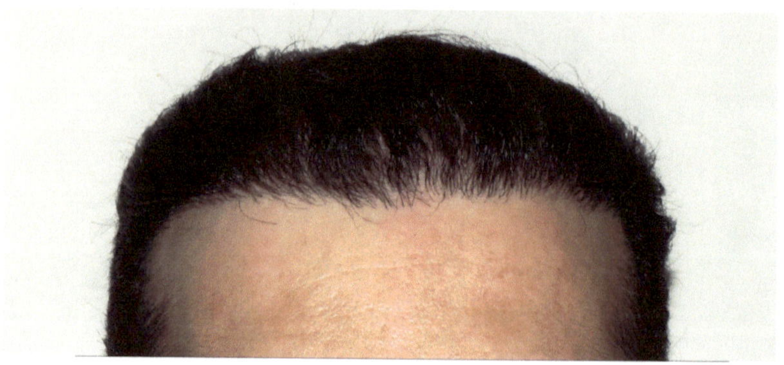

After 50 Weeks

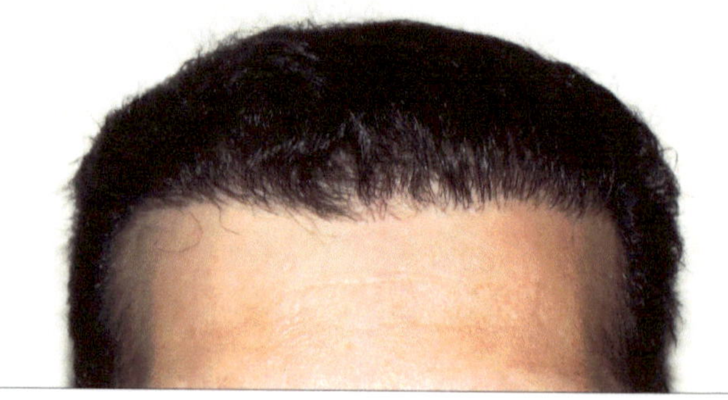

After 51 Weeks

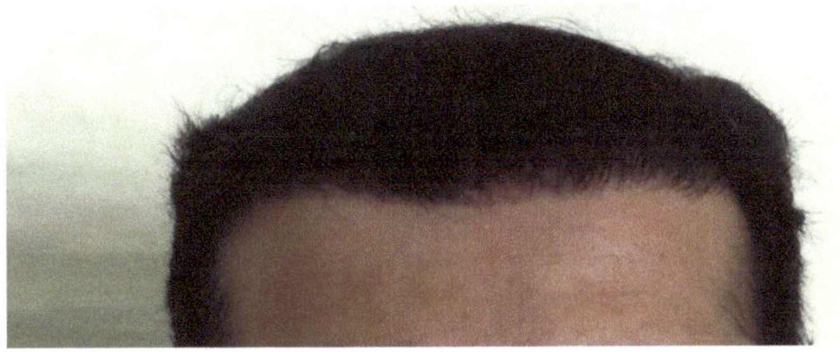

After 52 Weeks

The Final Photo

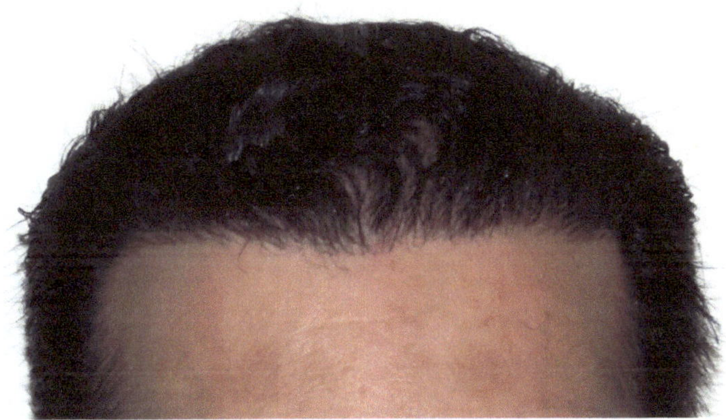

ABOUT THE AUTHOR

Brian Martin is a male located in Europe. He is an international performing artist who performs live shows on stage. He began noticing hair loss in his late twenties, at the beginning of the peak of his career. His hair continued to recede during the years that followed until he felt he had not other choice that to shave whatever hair he may have had at the time, and, go bald.

After many years of appearing on television and stage with a shaven head, Brian Martin still felt that appearance was important on stage and felt that hair completed the looked he aimed to have. With a choice between wearing a hairpiece or having a surgical procedure, he went for the latter.

After some research, he chose to have a FUE Hair Transplant in Turkey and found a company that dealt in this kind of tourism. Soon after his initial contacts and consultations. he ventured off for his life changing experience.

This book is a detailed account of his experience during the day of his transplant and the 6 days that followed.